Controlled Hypotension in Neuroanaesthesia

Controlled Hypotension in Neuroanaesthesia

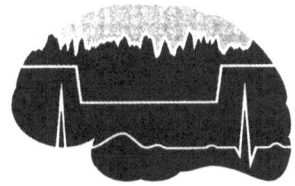

Edited by

D. Heuser
University of Tübingen
Tübingen, Federal Republic of Germany

D. G. McDowall
University of Leeds
Leeds, England

and

V. Hempel
University of Tübingen
Tübingen, Federal Republic of Germany

PLENUM PRESS • NEW YORK AND LONDON

Library of Congress Cataloging in Publication Data

Erwin Riesch Symposium (1981: Tübingen, Germany)
    Controlled hypotension in neuroanaesthesia.

    "Proceedings of an Erwin Riesch Symposium entitled Controlled hypotension in
neuroanaesthesia, held September 27–30, 1981, in Tübingen, Federal Republic of Ger-
many" – T.p. verso.
    Includes bibliographies and index.
    1. Brain – Surgery – Congresses. 2. Hypotension, Controlled – Congresses.
Anesthesia – Congresses. I. Heuser, D. II. McDowall, D. Gordon (David Gordon) III.
Hempel, Volker, IV. Title. [DNLM: 1. Brain – surgery – congresses. 2. Hypotension,
Controlled – congresses. WO 350 E73c 1981]
RD594.E75 1981   617′.481   85-6273
ISBN-13: 978-1-4612-9512-9   e-ISBN-13: 978-1-4613-2499-7
DOI: 10.1007/978-1-4613-2499-7

Proceedings of an Erwin Riesch Symposium entitled Controlled Hypotension in Neuroanaesthesia,
held September 27–30, 1981, in Tübingen, Federal Republic of Germany

©1985 Plenum Press, New York
Softcover reprint of the hardcover 1st edition 1985
A Division of Plenum Publishing Corporation
233 Spring Street, New York, N.Y. 10013

PREFACE

This book is based on the proceedings of a conference held in Tübingen, West Germany, in 1981, at which anesthesiologists, neuro-surgeons, pathologists and neurophysiologists met to consider the place of controlled hypotension in neurosurgery.

In the first part of the book alternative methods of inducing hypotension are considered, and it is important to emphasize that the techniques which are suitable for neurosurgery may not be so for other types of surgery, and vice versa. In neurosurgery, and par-ticularly in aneurysm surgery, the emphasis is on lowering intra-luminal pressure and not mainly on reducing blood flow or limiting tissue oozing. Another special consideration in neurosurgery is the influence of drugs used to induce hypotension on intracranial pressure, with nitroprusside (NTP), and especially nitroglycerine, increasing ICP in the closed skull and increasing brain "bulk" when the skull is open. These and other points are extensively covered.

The use of a non-essential technique like controlled hypotension demands that the procedure should carry minimal risk to the patient. Contributions in part IV consider the neuropathology associated with too severe a lowering of oxygen supply through hypotension. In the clinical avoidance of such ischemic changes in individual patients, monitoring of the brain electrical function is much the most import-ant and practical approach and is discussed in part III.

The Editors hope that the publication of these contributions to the Tübingen Symposium will help in the effective and safe appli-cation of the technique of controlled hypotension in neurosurgery.

The Editors

ACKNOWLEDGEMENTS

We gratefully acknowledge the financial support of the Symposium by the following companies:

Bayer AG
Boehringer Mannheim GmbH
B. Braun Melsungen AG
BYK – Gulden Lomberg
Glaxo Pharmazeutika GmbH
Hoechst AG
Immuno GmbH
Janssen GmbH
Dr F. Köhler Chemie GmbH
E. Lilly GmbH
E. Merck
Melusin-Schwarz GmbH
MSD Sharp & Dohme GmbH
Pfrimmer u. Co GmbH
Troponwerke GmbH & CoKG
UCB-Chemie GmbH
Winthrop GmbH
Zyma GmbH

CONTENTS

I

PHARMACOLOGICAL AND TOXICOLOGICAL ASPECTS OF
DRUGS USED FOR INDUCTION OF HYPOTENSION

Pharmacology of Drugs Used in Elective Hypotension
        for Neurosurgery   3
    P. Simpson

Specific Vascular Mechanisms of Hypotensive Acting
        Drugs   11
    T. Pasch

Rebound Arterial Hypertension Following Discontinuation
        of Sodium Nitroprusside: Aetiology and Prevention   21
    N. R. Fahmy

Is There Still Any Indication for Application of
        Volatile Anesthetics During Induction of
        Hypotension in Neurosurgery?   31
    G. Cunitz

Interactions of Anesthetic Drugs and Muscle Relaxants
        with Those Drugs Commonly Used for Controlled
        Hypotension   41
    V. Hempel and F. Münch

II
CEREBRAL BLOOD FLOW AND METABOLISM UNDER
CONDITIONS OF SYSTEMIC HYPOTENSION

Direct and Indirect Cerebral Effects of Deliberate
    Hypotension   49
    J. E. Cottrell

Autoregulation of Cerebral Blood Flow: Effects of
    Hypotensive Drugs   59
    W. Fitch, J. D. Pickard, D. I. Graham and
    I. Arendt

The Deleterious Effect of Excessive Tissue Lactic
    Acidosis in Brain Ischemia   63
    S. Rehncrona

Interaction Between Blood Glucose Level, Degree
    of Cerebral Tissue Acidosis and Cellular K^+
    Release Under Critical Cortical Flow Conditions   71
    D. Heuser, H. Guggenberger, H. Heinle and F. Braig

Controlled Hypotension in Neuroanesthesia   79
    P. J. Morris, D. Heuser and D. G. McDowall

Membrane Stabilization in the Ischemic Brain: A Mode
    of Protection?   85
    J. Astrup

Blood Flow and Oxidative Metabolism of the Young
    Adult and Aging Brain   93
    S. Hoyer

III
CEREBRAL ELECTRICAL ACTIVITY DURING SYSTEMIC
HYPOTENSION IN NEUROANESTHESIA

Electrical Monitoring of the Brain in Induced
    Hypotension - An Introduction to the Session   113
    D. G. McDowall

Critical Comparison of Monitoring EEG, Cerebral
    Function (CFM), Compressed Spectral Array (CSA)
    and Evoked Response Under Conditions of Reduced
    Cerebral Perfusion   117
    P. F. Prior

The Use of Somatosensory Evoked Potentials in
    Neurosurgical Practice   133
    L. Symon and A. D. J. Wang

Recent Aspects of Hypotensive Drug Effects on
     Intracranial Pressure   145
V. W. A. Pickerodt

IV
MORPHOLOGICAL ASPECTS OF CONTROLLED HYPOTENSION

The Neuropathology of Stagnant Hypoxia   157
D. I. Graham

Structural Changes in the Brain During Critical
     Reduction of Blood Flow or Oxygen Tension   171
H. Kalimo

The Significance of Low O_2 Tensions in the Brain
     Cortex for Occurrence of Metabolic Alterations
     Under Critical Flow Conditions   181
J. Grote, K. Zimmer and R. Schubert

V
CLINICAL ASPECTS OF CONTROLLED HYPOTENSION

Variations of the Instantaneous Heart Rate During
     Neuroleptanesthesia with Concomitant Continuous
     Infusions of Althesin and Sodium Nitroprusside   193
K. Huse and M. Krämer

Limitations of Induced Hypotension   203
U. Braun, J. Jansen, G. Rahlf and E. Turner

Pro and Contra Hypotension in Neurosurgery   211
E. Gordon

Chairman's Summary   219

List of Principal Contributors   223

Index   227

I

PHARMACOLOGICAL AND TOXICOLOGICAL ASPECTS OF
DRUGS USED FOR INDUCTION OF HYPOTENSION

PHARMACOLOGY OF DRUGS USED IN ELECTIVE

HYPOTENSION FOR NEUROSURGERY

P. J. Simpson

University Department of Anaesthetics
Royal Infirmary
Bristol BS2 8HW

INTRODUCTION

Although there has been much recent interest in the use of direct acting vasodilators in the production of elective hypotension for neurosurgery none of these is able to provide ideal hypotensive conditions in all cases. This is because of the wide variation in the type of hypotension required in different neurosurgical procedures. While some may require only moderate degrees of relatively prolonged hypotension others require instantaneous blood pressure control down to extremely low levels. In cases where the cerebral perfusion pressure is to be severely reduced it is essential to use drugs which allow the maintenance of autoregulation at these extremes.

The various agents and techniques available for the production of induced hypotension in neurosurgery are listed in Table 1. Although they will be considered as individual agents, their use is usually augmented by a moderate base-line hypotensive anaesthetic technique e.g. the avoidance of atropine premedication, the use of artificial ventilation to control carbon dioxide levels together with d-tubocurarine and a small dose of halothane or intravenous narcotic such as fentanyl or phenoperidine.

PHARMACOLOGICAL AGENTS USED IN ELECTIVE HYPOTENSION

Halothane

Although halothane produces a moderate degree of peripheral vasodilation, the overall fall in total peripheral resistance is of

3

Table 1. Drugs used in elective hypotension

Halothane ± curare and IPPV	
Ganglion Blockade	Hexamethonium
	Pentolinium
	Trimetaphan
α Blockade	Phenoxybenzamine
	Phentolamine
β Blockade	Propranolol
	Labetalol
	Practolol
Direct acting vasodilators	Sodium Nitroprusside
	Tri-nitro glycerine
Epidural or spinal anaesthesia	
(PEEP) and/or posture	

the order of 15-18 per cent. Vasodilation in the skin and splanchnic vascular beds is balanced by skeletal muscle vasoconstriction and any additional hypotension produced by halothane is as a direct result of myocardial depression. In addition the depressant effect of halothane both on the vagus nerve and on myocardial contraction tends to further reduce cardiac output. While halothane is often used successfully in low concentration as a background to hypotensive anaesthesia its use particularly in neurosurgery as a sole hypotensive agent in larger doses should be discouraged if the increase in intracranial pressure due to vasodilation is to be avoided.

Intermittent Positive Pressure Ventilation

Although not strictly pharmacological, the use of artificial ventilation in neurosurgery inevitably involves control of the arterial pCO_2 concentration. The pharmacological effects of excessively high or low carbon dioxide concentrations may have considerable influence on hypotension and bleeding since hypercapnia can produce vasodilation, hypertension and an increase in intracranial pressure while hypocapnia may result in vasoconstriction and cerebral ischaemia. The use of posture to augment the pharmacological effects of hypotensive agents is of considerable importance in neurosurgery particularly when used in conjunction with the ganglion blocking drugs. It is important to accurately measure systemic blood pressure at the level of the brain when employing a head-up tilt since a 25° inclination of the operating table will produce a difference in blood pressure between the brain and the heart of approximately 20mmHg.

Sympathetic Ganglionic Blockade
(Hexamethonium, Pentolinium, Trimetaphan, d-tubocurarine).

All these drugs produce autonomic ganglion blockade by competitive inhibition of acetylcholine. Their effects are not confined to sympathetic ganglia since acetylcholine transmission also occurs in the parasympathetic ganglia. Interruption of sympathetic outflow produces vasodilation which tends to be relatively slow in onset and recovery. The duration of hypotension produced by trimetaphan is relatively short (10-15 minutes) and for this reason the drug is often administered by intravenous infusion. In contrast a single injection of pentolinium produces hypotension for about 45 minutes and allows a slow return of blood pressure to normal values.

Although a number of gastrointestinal and urinary symptoms result from parasympathetic blockade the only two of clinical importance during hypotension are mydriasis and more important, tachycardia. The increase in heart rate which often accompanies induced hypotension produced by ganglion blockade may severely impair the effectiveness of these drugs in reducing bleeding. The tachyphylaxis which is particularly marked with triemtaphan may also make a stable blood pressure difficult to achieve.

Alpha Adrenergic Blockade
(Phentolamine, Phenoxybenzamine, Chloropromazine, Droperidol).

The alpha adrenergic blocking agents produce hypotension by competitive blockade of noradrenaline. While the effects of phentolamine are relatively short (20-40 minutes) and easily reversible, those of phenoxybenzamine may last several days since this drug forms an irreversible receptor complex. Phentolamine also exerts a direct myocardial stimulant effect, increasing both oxygen consumption and heart rate. Phenoxybenzamine may produce considerable sedation. While phentolamine is used in the rapid production of intraoperative vasodilation, phenoxybenzamine is more commonly employed for chronic vascular expansion prior to surgery to minimise the effects of circulating catecholamines e.g. in the surgical removal of phaeochromocytoma. Both chloropromazine and droperidol produce mild alpha adrenergic blockade which is often useful in the preoperative preparation of patients prior to hypotension and/or hypothermia.

β Adrenergic Blockade
(Propranolol, Practolol, Oxprenolol, Labethalol).

The main advantages of the β blocking drugs are in the reduction of heart rate and cardiac output. Many anaesthetists believe that the maintenance of a slow heart rate without any additional hypo-

tension often considerably reduces operative bleeding and propranolol
has often been used to produce this "rheostatic" hypotension. β
adrenergic blockade with either propranolol or oxprenolol is employed
both preoperatively and intraoperatively to counteract the tachycardia produced as a side effect of induced hypotension with either
ganglion blocking or direct acting vasodilatory drugs. In this
instance it would seem prudent to administer the drugs orally rather
than intravenously since this produces a steady intraoperative blood
level of the drug. Although the introduction of the combined α and
β adrenergic blocking drug labetalol appeared very promising it is
important to realize that the α blocking effects of the drug only
last for 30 minutes compared with a 90 minute duration of β blockade.
In addition the β blocking effects are five to seven times as potent
as the α blockade. The perioperative use of β blockade with either
propranolol or labetalol may have considerable benefit in the prevention of wide fluctuations in blood pressure particularly in
patients with subarachnoid haemorrhage and vasospasm.

Direct Acting Vasodilators
(Sodium nitroprusside, Trinitroglycerine)

     The recent interest in direct acting vasodilatory drugs began
with the reintroduction into clinical practice of sodium nitroprusside (SNP) in 1961. (Jones and Cole 1968). The main advantage of
this drug is in its extremely evanescent action, allowing rapid
reduction or restoration of blood pressure to hypotensive or normal
levels. It is the only drug capable of predictably producing "dial-
a-pressure" hypotension over relatively short periods e. g. in the
prevention of bleeding in meningiomas or to facilitate clipping of
cerebral aneurisms. As a vasodilator SNP inevitably produces an
increase in intracranial pressure and for this reason should probably
not be used with a closed cranium. Nevertheless autoregulation under
induced hypotension with nitroprusside is maintained at cerebral
perfusion pressures considerably lower than with other drugs. (Stoyka
and Schutz 1975). More recently trinitroglycerine (TNG) has been
advocated as a direct acting vasodilator for neurosurgery. (Chestnut
et al., 1978). Unlike sodium nitroprusside which dilates both resistance and capacitance vessels equally, nitroglycerine exerts its
effect principally upon the venous capacitance system. As a result
diastolic blood pressure is maintained at higher levels than with
nitroprusside and for this reason TNG may maintain coronary artery
perfusion more effectively than SNP. While this is probably of
little importance in fit patients it may be of considerable advantage
in patients with impaired myocardial or cerebral circulation. However the increase in intracranial pressure produced by nitroglycerine
may be even greater than with SNP.

TOXICITY OF SODIUM NITROPRUSSIDE

Shortly after the introduction of nitroprusside into clinical practice reports of fatalities due to drug administration were directly attributed to cyanide poisoning. (Jack 1974; Merrifield and Blundell 1974; Davies et al., 1975). Each molecule of sodium nitroprusside contains 5 cyanide radicals which are liberated on breakdown of the drug in either plasma or red blood cells. Several studies, however, have failed to demonstrate significant effects upon red cell oxygen transport of cyanide liberated during routine clinical use of nitroprusside. (Cailar et al., 1978; Vesey et al., 1980). The normal metabolic pathway of SNP breakdown is nonenzymatic, occurring in both red cells and plasma (Figure 1).

The intracellular reaction is catalyzed by the conversion of haemoglobin to methaemoglobin. Ultimately more than 98% of the cyanide produced from SNP is contained within the red blood cells while a small proportion is combined with either methaemoglobin or Vitamin B_{12}. The majority of cyanide is metabolised in the liver by the enzyme rhodanese to thiocyanate which is then excreted in the urine. Recent work has demonstrated that the rate limiting factor in cyanide metabolism is the availability of sulphydryl groups and that the administration of sodium thiosulphate can considerably enhance thiocyanate production and therefore the reduction of blood cyanide levels. (Krapez et al., 1981). The use of thiosulphate does not appear to affect the hypotension produced by nitroprusside. At the maximum safe doses recommended for nitroprusside administration ($1.5 mgkg^{1}$ (Vessey et al., 1975), or 10 $\mu gkg^{-1} min^{-1}$(Tinker and Michenfelder 1976), small increases in plasma lactate occur which are mirrored by increases in arterial base deficity. These changes are only minor, the maximum base deficit being of the order -6 to -7 mmols per litre and are spontaneously reversible on discontinuation of nitroprusside therapy. The routine measurement of acid-base balance during nitroprusside therapy would appear to provide adequate

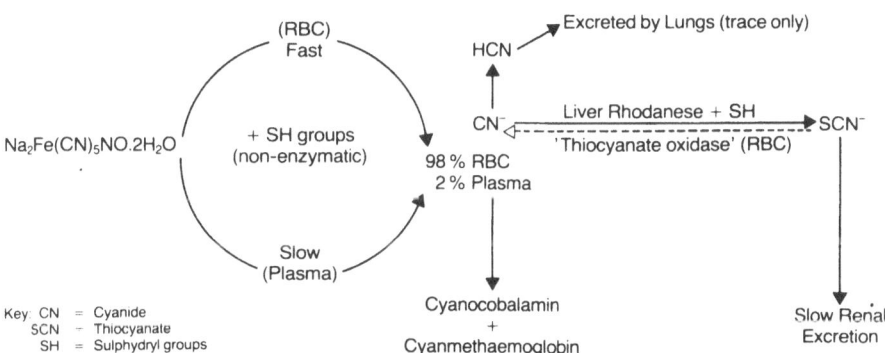

Fig. 1. Normal metabolic pathway of SNP breakdown.

clinical information of the development of cyanide toxicity during
routine clinical use.

In contrast to nitroprusside, nitroglycerine metabolism is not
potentially toxic. The trinitrate is hepatically metabolised by the
enzyme glutathione organic nitrate reductase through the dinitrate
and mononitrate to glycerol, although this occurs more slowly than
SNP metabolism. The dinitrate and mononitrate also possess mild
vasodilatory effects although this does not produce a clinical problem.

The clinically useful effects of nitroglycerine in contrast to
nitroprusside have been extensively studied (Michenfelder and Tinker
1977). Nitroglycerine produces a steadier and less dramatic reduction in arterial blood pressure, having a greater effect on systolic
than diastolic pressure and tending to maintain the blood flow.
Recovery from nitroglycerine-induced hypotension is also less rapid,
taking between 10 and 20 minutes in contrast to the 2-4 minutes with
SNP. It has been suggested that this slower effect of nitroglycerine
produces less overshoot of blood pressure either at induction of
hypotension or following restoration of normal blood pressure but as
the drug appears less effective in some cases in the production of
extreme hypotension its use may not be ideal in all forms of neurosurgery. In one study hypotension to 50mmHg was not possible in 3
out of 22 patients (Chestnut et al., 1978).

The use of sodium nitroprusside in patients already anaesthe-
tised with a background hypotensive anaesthetic technique would still
appear to be the agent of choice for the production of extreme hypotension for neurosurgery. No other drug at present provides the
predictable and rapid hypotensive effect necessary for many aspects
of intracranial surgery. Natural apprehension over the potential
toxicity of SNP has largely centered round a few reported cases all
of which were directly attributable to cyanide poisoning. Close
examination of these reports confirms that in all cases doses of SNP
vastly in excess of those required for routine clinical use were
needed to produce toxic symptoms. All drugs have a therapeutic ratio
and if this is exceeded symptoms of acute toxicity may occur. If the
dose of nitroprusside is limited to either $1.5mgkg^{-1}$ (Vessey et al.,
1975), or $10\mu gkg^{-1} min^{-1}$ (Tinker and Michenfelder 1976) toxic
symptoms will not occur in patients with normal renal and hepatic
function. For longer term infusion, in the presence of adequate
sulphydryl groups as the substrate for cyanide detoxification by
rhodanese, a maximum dose rate of 8 $\mu cgkg^{-1}$ (Michenfelder and Tinker
1977) has been shown to be satisfactory.

CONCLUSIONS

Despite the many and varied pharmacological methods available
for the reduction of sympathetic vascular tone there is no ideal

hypotensive agent for use in all circumstances. It is important for the anaesthetist and surgeon to determine whether the requirement is for a moderate degree of prolonged hypotension or a short period of severe hypotension and whether the hypotensive technique is being used to facilitate surgery by the reduction of operative bleeding or to make the impossible possible, while at the same time preventing the brain from serious hypoxic damage.

REFERENCES

Cailar, J. Du, Mathieu-Dande, J. C., Duschade J., Lamarche Y., and Castel, J., 1978, Nitroprusside, its metabolites and red cell function, Canadian Anaesthetists Society Journal, 25, 92-105.

Chestnut, J. S., Albin, M. S., Gonzalez-Abola, E., Newfield, P., and Maroon, J. C., 1978, Clinical evaluation of intravenous nitroglycerin for neurosurgery, Journal of Neurosurgery, 48, 704-711.

Davies, D. W., Kadar, D., Steward, D. J., and Munroe, I. R., 1975, A sudden death associated with the use of sodium nitroprusside for the induction of hypotension during anaesthesia, Canadian Anaesthetists Society Journal, 22, 547-552.

Jack, R., 1974, The toxicity of sodium nitroprusside, British Journal of Anaesthesia, 46, 952.

Jones, G., and Cole, P. V., 1968, Sodium nitroprusside as a hypotensive agent, British Journal of Anaesthesia, 40, 804.

Krapez, J. R., Vesey, C. J., Adams, L., and Cole, P. W., 1981, Effects of cyanide antidotes used with sodium nitroprusside infusion: sodium thiosulphate and hydroxocobalamin given prophylactically to dogs, Brit.J.Anaes., 53, 793-804.

Merrifield, A., and Blundell, M., 1974, Toxicity of sodium nitroprusside, British Journal of Anaesthesia, 46, 324.

Michenfelder, J. D., and Tinker, J. H., 1977, Cyanide toxicity and thiosulphate protection during chronic administration of sodium nitroprusside in the dog., Anesthesiology, 47, 441-448.

Stoyka, W. W., and Schutz, H., 1975, The cerebral response to sodium nitroprusside and trimetaphan controlled hypotension, Canadian Anaesthetists Society Journal, 22, 275-282.

Tinker, J. H., and Michenfelder, J. D., 1976, Sodium nitroprusside; Pharmacology, Toxicology and Sodium Therapeutics, Anesthesiology, 45, 340-354.

Vessey, C. J., Cole, P. V., and Simpson, J. P., 1975, Sodium nitroprusside in anaesthesia, British Medical Journal, 3, 229.

Vessey, C. J., Krapez, J. R., and Cole, P. V., 1980, The effects of sodium nitroprusside and cyanide on haemoglobin function, J.Pharm.Pharmacol., 32, 256-261.

SPECIFIC VASCULAR MECHANISMS OF HYPOTENSIVE ACTING DRUGS

T. Pasch

Department of Anaesthesiology
University of Erlangen-Nuremberg
D- 8520 Erlangen
Federal Republic of Germany

In vitro, the demonstration of the relaxant effect of a pharmacological drug depends on a certain degree of activation of the vascular smooth muscle cells (van Nueten and Wellens 1979).

Only a few blood vessels on which experiments of this sort can be carried out manifest adequate spontaneous activity. Other vascular preparations representing the main sites of action of hypotensive acting drugs, first have to be constricted by applying suitable stimuli before a drug-induced dilation can be triggered and studied in detail.

In principle, the process of triggering a contraction is identical for all vascular smooth muscle cells. For the interaction between actin and myosin filaments an increase in the concentration of free cytoplasmic calcium ions (Ca^{2+}) is a prerequisite. This is achieved by a change in the polarization and permeability of the cell membrane. Such a change can be brought about by the intrinsic activity of the cell membrane or the binding of a vasoactive substance to the membrane. The increase in membrane permeability results in an influx of extracellular Ca^{2+}; in addition, Ca^{2+} is also released from intracellular stores. The result is an increase in the concentration of intracellular Ca^{2+} (activator-Ca^{2+}). If the amount of available activator-Ca^{2+} exceeds a given threshold concentration, the interaction between actin and myosin filaments is triggered and the cell contracts (van Breemen et al., 1980; Vanhoutte 1978).

In its details, the Ca^{2+} -dependent mechanism responsible for activating the actomyosin system in smooth muscle does not appear completely identical with that found in striated muscle (Cheung 1980;

11

Hartshorne 1980; Johansson 1981; Keatinge and Harman 1980). Contraction is terminated or inhibited if inhibitory substances become effective or when the triggering process (myogenic activity or stimulatory substance) stops. Then the sarcoplasmic activator-Ca^{2+} drops below the threshold concentration by being trapped again into intracellular stores, probably sarcoplasmic reticulum (van Breemen et al., 1980), or by being expelled into the extracellular space.

All drugs with a vasodilatory action exert their effects on the process of Ca^{2+} control of the actomyosin complex. Irrespective of the considerable variation that exists among various species, various blood vessels, and also among the various possibilities of activating smooth muscle cells, vasodilators can become effective in either of two ways. When they inhibit the release or the receptor-binding of vasoconstrictive agonists, they behave as inhibitors of vasoconstriction, and this manifests as a vasodilation. If they have a direct inhibitory effect on the availability of activator-Ca^{2+}, they may be termed true vasodilating drugs. Such a differentiation has not found general acceptance (van Nueten and Wellens 1979), but, for the discussion here, it is of didactic usefulness. This article describes the modes of action of such drugs as are employed intraoperatively to reduce arterial blood pressure. We cannot deal here systematically with substances used to treat arterial hypertensive disease.

INHIBITORS OF VASOCONSTRICTION

The most important of the physiological vasoconstrictors are the catecholamines and angiotensin II. The most important of the catecholamines is noradrenaline, which reaches the vascular wall either via the circulating blood, or via the sympathetic nerve endings. Its action can be blocked by inhibition of its release (indirect) or by blocking the receptor on the membrane of the smooth muscle cell (direct). Of therapeutic importance for induced intraoperative hypotension are the ganglionic blockers, substances that inhibit the release of noradrenaline, and the alpha-adrenergic antagonists (Figure 1).

Ganglionic blocking agents as trimethaphan and pentolinium stabilize the postsynaptic membrane against the effects of acetylcholine that is released at the preganglionic nerve endings (Volle and Koelle 1975). In the last instance, the result of this is to prevent the release of noradrenaline at the neuroeffector junction, and vasodilation occurs. Among the numerous substances that block the liberation of noradrenaline from the postganglionic nerve terminals halothane might be mentioned in view of its intraoperative application. Results of Muldoon et al., may be interpreted to mean that halothane inhibits the release of noradrenaline by the nerve endings, without impairing the response of the smooth muscle cell to endogenous or exogenous noradrenaline.

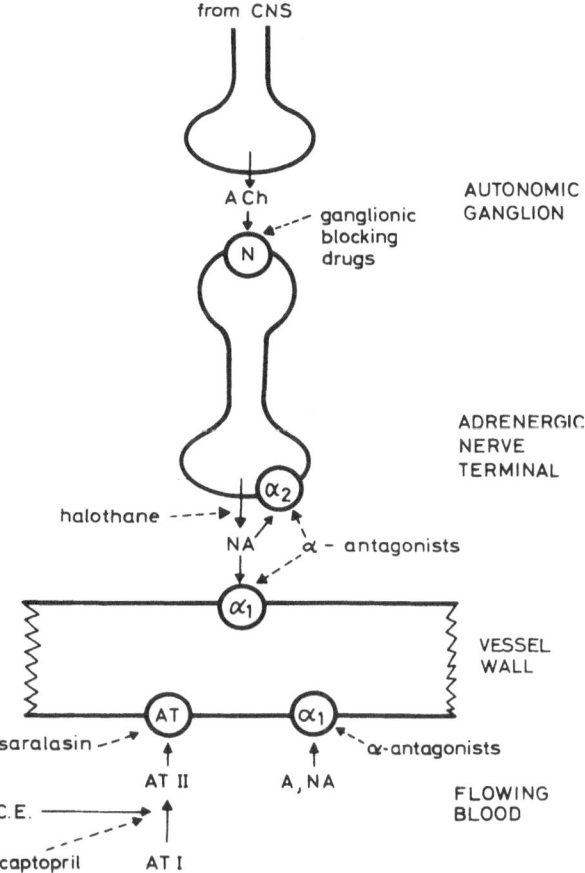

Fig. 1. Schematic representation of vasodilatation by inhibition of vasoconstrictor agonists. A = adrenaline; NA = noradrenaline; ACh = acetylcholine; AT = angiotensin; N = nicotinic receptor; α = alpha-adrenoceptor; C. E. = converting enzyme.

Occupancy of alpha-receptor sites on the postsynaptic membrane prevents noradrenaline from binding to the receptor and thus brings about the dilation of the blood vessel. From among the category of alpha-adrenergic antagonists, phentolamine and urapidil may be considered for use in surgery to lower blood pressure. In recent years, a mass of findings has been accumulated showing that there are two different subtypes of alpha-adrenergic receptors in existence (Hoffmann and Lefkowitz 1980; Langer 1977; Starke 1981).

As is well known, stimulation of the postjunctional alpha-receptors leads to constriction of smooth muscle cells. In addition, there are also alpha-receptors on the presynaptic membrane of the

nerve endings themselves (prejunctional alpha-receptors). If they
are stimulated by noradrenaline, the amount of noradrenaline released
by the action of nerve impulses, is reduced. Thus, high concentrations of noradrenaline in the synaptic gap have the effect of
reducing the amount of noradrenaline released by subsequent nerve
impulses. Postsynaptic receptors are referred to as $alpha_1$-, presynaptic as $alpha_2$-receptors. These two receptor subtypes are vari-
ously stimulated by agonists and antagonists. Thus, phentolamine
acts with equal intensity both on $alpha_1$- and $alpha_2$-receptors, and
this is thought to be, in part, responsible for its side-effects such
as tachycardia and inotropic influence on the myocardium (Hoffmann
and Lefkowitz 1980). The picture is complicated further by the fact
that there are also postjunctional $alpha_2$-receptors and that the
distribution of the subtypes in vascular muscles from different sites
varies considerably (DeMay and Vanhoutte 1981; Sullivan and Drew
1980).

     Inhibitory effects similar to those exerted on noradrenaline can
also be exerted on angiotensin II using pharmacological drugs (Miller
1981). The conversion of the biologically largely ineffective angiotensin I to angiotensin II can be prevented by inhibitors of the
converting enzyme (captopril, teprotide), The angiotensin receptor
in the vascular wall can be inactivated by occupying it with an
analogue of angiotensin II (saralasin). At present, however, angiotensin antagonism has no significance for intraoperative lowering of
blood pressure.

DIRECT VASODILATORS

     Direct vasodilators prevent an increase in activator-Ca^{2+}. For
the sake of simplicity, they may be classed into four groups (Figure
2). Ca-antagonists, which include verapamil, nifedipine, cinnarizine
and flunarizine, reduce the permeability of the membrane for Ca^{2+},
that is, they reduce the influx of extracellular Ca^{2+}, so that not
enough activator-Ca^{2+} is available (Fleckenstein 1977; van Nueten and
Wollens 1979). Among the above-mentioned substances, there are
marked differences in the selectivity of their action on various
preparations and with different types of activation (Broekaert and
Godfraind 1979; Mikkelsen et al., 1979; Triggle and Swamy 1980; van
Nueten et al., 1980). Beta-adrenergic agonists exert their relaxant
effect by hyperpolarizing the cell membrane and elevating the intracellular cAMP concentration due to activation of the adenylate cyc-
lase within the membrane (Bevan et al., 1978; Keatinge and Harmann
1980). Yet another group of vasodilators, the inhibitors of phos-
phodiesterase, increase the concentration of intracellular cAMP. To
this group belong papavarine and theophylline (Ferrari 1974). It is
probable that papavarine additionally acts as a Ca-antagonist
(Broekaert and Godfraind 1979; Thorens and Haeusler 1979).

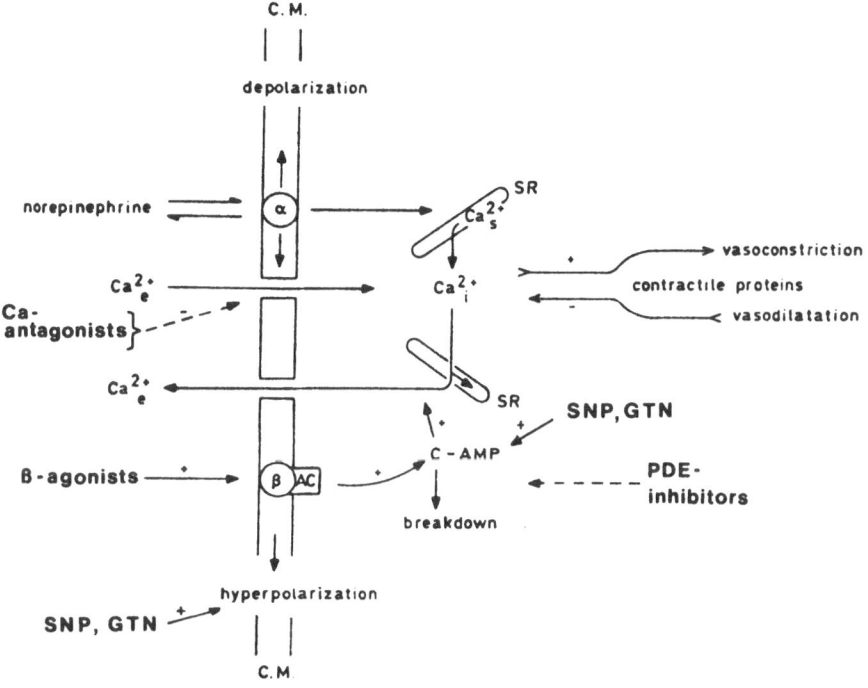

Fig. 2.   Schematic representation of mechanisms of direct vasodilata-
          tion.   C. M. = membrane of vascular smooth muscle cell; SR =
          sarcoplasmic reticulum ; e = extracellular; i = intracellu-
          lar; s = stored; AC = adenylate cyclase; α, β = alpha- and
          beta-adrenoceptors; PDE = phosphodiesterase; SNP = sodium
          nitroprusside; GTN = glyceryl trinitrate. Modified after
          van Nueten and Wellens (37) and reproduced by permission of
          the authors and the Angiology Research Foundation.

     The vasodilators most commonly employed for controlling blood
pressure during surgery are sodium nitroprusside (SNP) and glyceryl
trinitrate (GTN).   They have powerful relaxant effects on vascular
smooth muscle and do not interact with adrenergic or cholinergic
receptors (Kreye et al., 1975; Verhaege and Sheperd 1976).   There are
clearly recognizable differences between these two substances.   The
well known fact, seen in clinical experience and in experimental
results, that SNP has a more powerful relaxing effect on the arteriolar resistance vessels than does GTN, while GTN has a greater
dilatory effect on the venous capacitance vessels (Collier et al.,
1978; Miller et al., 1976) can also be demonstrated in vitro (Bevan
et al., 1978; Kreye et al., 1975; Thorens and Haeusler 1979; Verhaege
and Sheperd 1976).   This difference in the behavior of these two
vasodilators can, in part, be traced back to the - admittedly largely
hypothetical - mode of action.

SNP has no influence on the influx of Ca^{2+} (Thorens and Haeusler 1979; Verhaege and Shepherd 1976; Zsotér et al., 1977) and, under suitable experimental conditions, even eliminates residual constrictions following the action of Ca-antagonists (Golenhofen 1978; Triggle and Swamy 1980). In contrast, high concentrations of GTN can, to a limited extent, inhibit Ca^{2+} influx (Fleckenstein 1977; Thorens and Haeusler 1979; Zsotér et al., 1974). There is evidence that catecholamine-induced constrictions of arteriolar vessels are independent of extracellular Ca^{2+}, in contrast to constrictions produced in the venules (Altura 1978). These various results may be interpreted to mean that SNP reduces the amount of activator-Ca^{2+} completely independently of extracellular Ca^{2+}, and for this reason has a marked relaxant effect on arterioles. In contrast, GTN possibly inhibits the influx of Ca^{2+} in addition to its intracellular site of action and thus exerts a greater action on capacitance vessels than does SNP. A further in vitro difference between these two drugs concerns their influence on the ^{45}Ca uptake by subcellular fractions of rabbit aorta (Thorens and Haeusler 1979). At high doses, which also inhibit the influx of ^{45}Ca, GTN blocks the uptake in fractions both of the endoplasmic reticulum and the plasma membrane, while SNP is ineffective. Whether this blockade of the intracellular Ca^{2+} accumulation has any significance for the relaxant effect of GTN, however, is not yet known.

Not all experimental results suggest a different mode of action for GTN and SNP (Fermum et al., 1977; Kukovetz et al., 1979). Low concentrations of SNP hyperpolarize the cell membrane (Haeusler and Thorens 1976) which, in the case of the beta-adrenergic agonists, contributes to the relaxant effect (Figure 2). The investigations of Kreye suggest that a reduction in the Cl^- conductivity of the cell membrane which can be brought about both by SNP and GTN, is the cause of the hyperpolarization. At higher doses, it is probable that SNP and GTN permeate the membrane and exert an intracellular action on the Ca^{2+}-dependent regulation of the actin-myosin reaction (Fermum et al., 1977), as will be described below. Measurements of the ^{45}Ca efflux carried out by Zsotér et al., have shown that it is increased both by GTN (Zsotér et al., 1979) and by SNP (Zsotér et al., 1977). Accordingly, both substances appear to lower the concentration of activator-Ca^{2+} by promoting the elimination of Ca^{2+} from the cell. In contrast, Hester et al. (1979), have found an inhibition of ^{45}Ca-efflux and interpreted this to mean that SNP increases the retention of Ca^{2+} at noradrenaline-sensitive sites of the cell membrane. This, too, would result in a lowering of the concentration of free activator-Ca^{2+}. There is, however, evidence that relaxation is effected by Ca^{2+} accumulation by an intracellular Ca^{2+} pool different from that which releases Ca^{2+} during activation (van Breemen et al., 1980).

Recently, a number of general theories of the actions of vasodilators have been developed, but further experimental results are

really needed. For this reason, these theories are only briefly
outlined here. Ethacrynic acid which alkylates sulfhydryl (SH)
groups, blocks the greater part of the response of rabbit thoracic
aortic strips to a number of vasodilating drugs, e.g. GTN, SNP,
isoproterenol, papaverine. On the basis of these findings, the
working hypothesis has been developed that some vasodilators interact
with more or less specific receptor sites within the membrane by
oxidizing SH groups and that, besides specific receptors, all vasodilators may act via a common intermediate reaction involving SH
groups in the tissue (Needleman et al., 1973).

There is evidence that GTN and SNP increase the intracellular
concentration of cyclic nucleotides, which then trigger the relaxation process. Whether cAMP (Andersson 1973; van Breemen et al.,
1980), cGMP (Böhme et al., 1978; Burkhard 1977; Diamond 1978;
Gruetter et al., 1981; Kukovetz et al., 1979), or both nucleotides
together effect relaxation, is not yet known (Keatinge and Harmann
1980). It has been shown that cAMP blocks and Ca^{2+} activates the
enzyme myosin light-chain kinase (MLCK), which executes the phosphorylation of the 20,000 dalton myosin light chain. This reaction
is thought to be the crucial step in the formation of the actomyosin
complex ((Johannson 1981). The MLCK was found to be composed of two
subunits, the smaller being identified as the Ca^{2+}-binding protein
calmodulin (Hartshorne 1980), which is involved in a large number of
enzymic mechanisms (Cheung 1980). Furthermore, the smooth muscle
contains a phosphatase capable of dephosphorylating the myosin. The
action of this enzyme results in the dissociation of the actomyosin
and the relaxation of the smooth muscle cell (Hartshorne 1980).
Hence, it is certainly a possibility that vasodilators may activate
this enzyme or, more probably, prevent the binding of Ca^{2+} to calmodulin and thus inhibit the MLCK, without exerting any direct influence on the intracellular concentration of free Ca^{2+} (Keatinge and
Harmann 1980).

REFERENCES

Altura, B. M., 1978, Pharmacology of venular smooth muscle: new
    insights, Microvasc.Res., 16, 91.
Andersson, R., 1973, Cyclic AMP as a mediator of the relaxing action
    of papaverine, nitroglycerine, diazoxide and hydralazine in
    intestinal and vascular smooth muscle, Acta Pharmacol.
    Toxicol., 32, 321.
Bevan, J. A., Pegram, B. L., Prehn, J. L., Winquist, R. J., 1978,
    β-adrenergic receptor-mediated vasodilatation, in: "Mechanisms
    of Vasodilatation," P. M. Vanhoutte, I. Leusen, eds., p. 258,
    Karger, Basel.
Böhme, E., Graf, H., Schultz, G., 1978, Effects of sodium nitroprus-
    side and other smooth muscle relaxants on cyclic GMP formation
    in smooth muscle and platelets, Adv.Cycl.Nucl.Res., 9, 131.

Broekaert, A., Godfraind, T., 1979,: A comparison of the inhibitory
    effect of cinnarizine and papaverine on the noradrenaline- and
    calcium-evoked contraction of isolated rabbit aorta and mesen-
    teric arteries, Eur.J.Pharmacol., 53, 281.
Burkard, W. R., 1977, Effect of sodium nitroprusside on contractile
    state and cyclic nucleotide levels in rabbit arteries.
    Naunyn-Schmiedeberg's Arch.Pharmacol., 297, R12.
Cheung, W. Y., 1980, Calmodulin plays a pivotal role in cellular
    regulation, Science, 207, 19.
Collier, J. G., Lorge, R. E., Robinson, B. F., 1978: Comparison of
    effects of tolmesoxide (RX 71107), diazoxide, hydrallazine,
    prazosin, glyceryl trinitrate and sodium nitroprusside on
    forearm arteries and dorsal hand veins of man, Brit.J.Clin.
    Pharmacol., 5, 35.
De May, J., Vanhoutte, P. M., 1981: Uneven distribution of post-
    junctional alpha$_1$ - and alpha$_2$ -like adrenoceptors in canine
    arterial and venous smooth muscle, Circ.Res., 48, 875.
Diamond, J., 1978, Role of cyclic nucleotides in control of smooth
    muscle contraction, Adv.Cycl.Nucl.Res., 9, 327.
Fermum, R., Meisel, P., Klinner, U., 1977, Versuche zum Wirkungs-
    mechanismus von Gefäßspasmolytika. 3. Wirkung von Nitro-
    prussid-Natrium, Nitroglycerin, Prenylamin und Verapamil an
    der Fluorid-induzierten Kontraktur isolierter Koronararterien.
    Acta Biol.Med.Germ., 36, 245.
Ferrari, M., 1974, Effects of papaverine on smooth muscle and their
    mechanisms, Pharmacol.Res.Comm., 6, 97.
Fleckenstein, A., 1977, Specific pharmacology of calcium in
    myocardium cardiac pacemakers, and vascular smooth muscle,
    Ann.Rev.Phamacol.Toxicol., 17, 149.
Golenhofen, K., 1978, Die myogene Basis der glattmuskulären Motorik,
    Klin.Wochenschr., 56, 211.
Gruetter, C. A., Kadowitz, P. J., Ignarro, L. J., 1981, Methylene
    blue inhibits coronary arterial relaxation und guanylate
    cyclase activation by nitro-glycerin, sodium nitrite, and amyl
    nitrite, Can.J.Physiol.Pharmacol., 59, 150.
Haeusler, G., Thorens, S., 1976, The pharmacology of vaso-active
    antihypertensives, in: "Vascular Neuroeffector Mechanisms," J.
    A. Bevan, G. Burnstock, B. Johansson, R. A. Maxwell, O. A.
    Nedergaard, eds., p. 232, Karger, Basel.
Hartshorne, D. J., 1980, Biochemical basis for contraction of vas-
    cular smooth muscle, Chest 78 (Suppl.), 140.
Hester, R. K., Weiss, G. B., Fry, W. J., 1979, Differing actions of
    nitroprusside and D-600 on tension and ^{45}Ca fluxes in canine
    renal arteries, J.Pharmacol.Exp.Ther., 208, 155.
Hoffmann, B. B., Lefkowitz, R. J., 1980, Alpha-adrenergic subtypes,
    New Engl.J.Med., 302, 1390.
Johansson, B., 1981, Vascular smooth muscle reactivity, Ann.Rev.
    Physiol., 43, 359.
Keatinge, W. R., Harman, M. C., 1980, "Local Mechanisms Controlling
    Blood Vessels," Academic Press, London.

Kreye, V. A. W., 1978, Organic nitrates, sodium nitroprusside, and
    vasodilation, in "Mechanisms of Vasodilatation," P. M.
    Vanhoutte, I. Leusen, eds., p. 158, Karger, Basel.
Kreye, V. A. W., Baron, G. D., Lüth, J. B., Schmidt-Gayk, H., 1975:
    Mode of action of sodium nitroprusside on vascular smooth
    muscle. Naunyn-Schmiedeberg's Arch.Pharmacol., 288, 381.
Kukovetz, W. R., Holzmann, S., Wurm, A., Pöch, G., 1979, Evidence for
    cyclic GMP-mediated effects of nitro-compounds in coronary
    smooth muscle, Naunyn-Schmiedeberg's Arch.Pharmacol., 310,
    129.
Langer, S. Z., 1977, Presynaptic receptors and their role in the
    regulation of transmitter release, Brit.J.Pharmacol., 60, 481.
Mikkelsen, E., Andersson, K.-E., Lederballe-Pedersen, O., 1979:
    Verapamil and nifedipine inhibition of contractions induced by
    potassium and noradrenaline in human mesenteric arteries and
    veins, Acta Pharmacol.Toxicol., 44, 110.
Miller, E. D., 1981, The role of the renin-angiotensin-aldosterone
    system in circulatory control and in hypertension, Brit.J.
    Anaesth., 53, 711.
Miller, R. R., Vismara, L. A., Williams, D. O., Amsterdam, E. A.,
    Mason, D. T., 1976, Pharmacological mechanisms for left vent-
    ricular unloading in clinical congestive heart failure.
    Differential effects of nitroprusside, phentolamine, and
    nitroglycerin on cardiac function and peripheral circulation,
    Circulation 39, 127.
Muldoon, S. M., Vanhoutte, P. M., Lorenz, R. R., van Dyke, R. A.,
    1975, Venomotor changes caused by halothane acting on the
    sympathetic nerves, Anesthesiology, 43, 41.
Needleman, P., Jakschik, B. A., Johnson, E. M., 1973, Sulfhydryl
    requirement for relaxation of vascular smooth muscle, J.
    Pharmacol.Exp.Ther., 187, 324.
Starke, K., 1981, α-adrenoceptor subclassification, Rev.Physiol.Bio.
    chem.Pharmacol., 88, 199.
Sullivan, A. T., Drew, G. M., 1980, Pharmacological characterization
    of pre- and postsynaptic α-adrenoceptors in dog saphenous
    vein, Naunyn Schmiedeberg's Arch.Pharmacol., 314, 249.
Thorens, S., Haeusler, G., 1979, Effects of some vasodilators on
    calcium translocation in intact and fractionated vascular
    smooth muscle, Eur.J.Pharmacol., 54, 79.
Triggle, D. J., Swamy, V. C., 1980, Pharmacology of agents that
    affect calcium, Agonists and antagonists, Chest 78 (Suppl.),
    174.
van Breemen, C., Aaronson, P., Loutzenhiser, R., Meisheri, K., 1980,
    Ca^{2+} movements in smooth muscle, Chest 78 (Suppl.), 157.
Vanhoutte, P. M., 1978, Heterogeneity in vascular smooth muscle, in:
    "Microcirculation," G. Kaley, B. M. Altura, eds., vol. 2, p.
    181, University Park Press, Baltimore.
van Nueten, J. M., van Beek, J., Janssen, P. A. J., 1978, The vas-
    cular effects of flunarizine as compared with those of other
    clinically used vasoactive substances, Arzneimittelforsch.,
    28, 2082.

van Nueten, J. M., Wellens, D., 1979, Mechanisms of vasodilatation
    and antivasoconstriction, <u>Angiology</u> 30, 440.
Verhaeghe, R. H., Shepherd, J. T., 1976, Effect of nitroprusside on
    smooth muscle and adrenergic nerve terminals in isolated blood
    vessels, <u>J.Pharmacol.Exp.Ther.</u>, 199, 269.
Volle, R. L., Koelle, G. B., 1975, Ganglionic stimulating and block-
    ing agents, <u>in</u> "The Pharmacological Basis of Therapeutics, 5th
    ed.," L. S. Goodman, A. Gilman, eds., p. 565, Macmillan, New
    York.
Zsotér, T. T., Henein, N. F. Wolchinsky, C., The effect of sodium
    nitroprusside on the uptake and efflux of ^{45}Ca from rabbit and
    rat vessels, <u>Eur.J.Pharmacol.</u>, 45, 7.
Zsotér, T. T., Jacyk, P., Wolchinsky, C., 1974, The effect of
    vasodilators on calcium kinetics in blood vessels,
    <u>Arch.Intern.Pharmacodyn.Ther.</u>, 212, 328.

REBOUND ARTERIAL HYPERTENSION FOLLOWING DISCONTINUATION

OF SODIUM NITROPRUSSIDE: AETIOLOGY AND PREVENTION

N. R. Fahmy

Harvard Medical School
Massachusetts General Hospital
Boston, MA 02114, USA

Adverse hemodynamic reactions are known to occur after abrupt withdrawal of cardiovascular drugs (Gerber and Nies, 1979). We and others (Khambata et al., 1979; Packer et al., 1979) have observed that the cessation of sodium nitroprusside (SNP) infusion was followed by an increase in arterial blood pressure. This rebound hypertension can be hazardous when nitroprusside is employed to decrease preload and afterload in patients with severe chronic heart failure or to control arterial pressure for repair of cerebral aneurysms or other vascular lesions. The renin-angiotension system is involved in this phenomenon. The present study was designed (1) to characterize the changes in hemodynamics, plasma catecholamines and plasma renin activity that follow the abrupt cessation of nitroprusside infusion for controlled intraoperative hypotension and (2) to determine the effects of pretreatment with intravenous propranolol on these nitroprusside-induced changes.

MATERIALS AND METHODS

Sixteen patients whose ages ranged from 18 to 59 years were studied with their consent. There were 9 males and 7 females, and their weights ranged from 54 to 78 Kg. None of these patients had clinical evidence of cardiopulmonary, hepatic, renal or electrolyte disorder, and none was receiving any medication. All patients were maintained on a regular diet with a normal sodium intake. All patients were scheduled for major orthopedic procedures. The patients were divided into two groups. Group 1 consisted of the first ten consecutive patients and they received nitroprusside. Group 2 consisted of six patients who were pretreated with intravenous propranolol, 0.05 mg/kg, before nitroprusside administration.

21

The anesthetic management of all patients was similar. Pre-medication consisted of diazepam, 10 mg orally, one hour before anesthetic induction. Thiopentone was given for induction of anes-thesia, in a dose of 5 mg/kg. This was followed by succinylcholine, 1 mg/kg, to facilitate endotracheal intubation. Anesthesia was maintained with halothane 1% inspired concentration, nitrous oxide-oxygen, 60:40%, and curare, 0.4 mg/kg. Ventilation was controlled mechanically to maintain arterial PCO_2 between 35 and 40 mm Hg. In Group 2 patients, propranolol, 0.05 mg/kg, was given slowly intra-venously before the induction of anesthesia. Sodium nitroprusside infusion was used to decrease mean arterial pressure between 50 and 55 mm Hg by regulating the infusion rate. All patients received lactated Ringer's solution at the rate of 4 ml/kg/hr. Colloids, in the form of packed erythrocytes and 5% human albumin, were admin-istered to replace blood loss which was measured by weighing sponges and suction losses.

Eight sets of measurements were made: before induction of anes-thesia; before the start of nitroprusside-induced hypotension; 30 minutes after hypotension was begun, before and 5, 15, 30 and 60 minutes after discontinuation of nitroprusside. Each set of obser-vations included measurement of cardiac output (dye-dilution), arterial and right atrial pressure (Statham pressure transducers), heart rate (electrocardiogram), arterial blood PO_2, PCO_2, and pH (standard electrodes). In addition, plasma renin activity (PRA) was determined by radioimmunoassay of generated angiotensin I according to Sealey et al. (1972), plasma catecholamines were assayed with a modification of the method of Peuler and Johnson (1977), and plasma electrolytes were determined by flame photometry. Systemic vascular resistance and stroke volume were derived from standard formulae (Fahmy and Laver, 1976).

Oesophegeal temperature was measured with a thermistor probe; body temperature was maintained constant by adjusting ambient tem-perature and humidifying inspired gases.

A two-way analysis of variance was employed to test whether the variables, measured and derived, changed over time. Comparisons were computed by Student's t tests; $P < 0.05$ was considered significant. All values are given as mean ± SEM.

RESULTS

There were no significant differences between the two groups with regard to age, sex, awake hemodynamic variables and awake plasma catecholamines and PRA.

Hemodynamic Variables (Table 1)

In both groups of patients, halothane N_2O-O_2 anesthesia for 30 to 45 minutes produced a significant decrease ($P < 0.05$) in mean arterial pressure and cardiac output. Systemic vascular resistance showed a small insignificant increase. Right arterial pressure increased significantly in Group 1 patients only.

Infusion of sodium nitroprusside was associated with significant decreases in mean arterial pressure, systemic vascular resistance and mean right atrial pressure in Group 1 patients. Cardiac output increased significantly (from 3.8 ± 0.3 to 4.8 ± 0.4) due to an increase in heart rate and stroke volume. In Group 2 patients, mean arterial blood pressure and systemic vascular resistance decreased significantly. Cardiac output, heart rate, mean right atrial pressure and stroke volume were not changed with SNP infusion.

Upon cessation of SNP administration, Group 1 patients exhibited important hemodynamic changes which were most marked after 15 minutes and subsided after 30 minutes. Mean arterial pressure increased due to a significant increase in systemic vascular resistance; a decrease in cardiac output occurred. These changes returned to preinfusion values after 30 minutes.

In Group 2 patients, however, mean arterial blood pressure and other hemodynamic variables returned gradually to preinfusion values.

Thus, pretreatment with propranolol prevented hemodynamic events that followed withdrawal of SNP.

Plasma Renin Activity and Catecholamines (Table 2)

General anesthesia produced a decrease in arterial blood pressure which was associated with an increase in plasma renin activity in Group 1 only. Plasma norepinephrine, epinephrine and dopamine levels did not change in either group.

Infusion of SNP was associated with significant increases in PRA and catecholamines ($P < 0.001$). These changes were prevented by pretreatment with propranolol in Group 2 patients.

In Group 1, following discontinuation of SNP administration, PRA was still significantly elevated above preinfusion values. Plasma catecholamines were significantly higher than both pre-infusion and pre-SNP withdrawal values. These biogenic amines were high for 15 minutes and returned to preinfusion values between 30 to 60 minutes. In patients pretreated with propranolol, no significant changes were observed after cessation of SNP infusion.

Table 1. Hemodynamic data before, during and after sodium nitroprusside infusion in ten (Group I) patients (first line in each panel) and in six (Group II) patients (second line in each panel) who were given intravenous propranolol (0.05 mg/kg) before nitroprusside infusion.

	Before Hypotension		30 min after hypotension	Before	Discontinuation of nitroprusside Minutes after			
	Awake	Hypotension			5	15	30	60
Mean arterial pressure mmHg	98±4	86±6	54±3	55±4	94±9	97±8	84±5	83±4
	95±4	82±3	53±2	52±3	69±5	78±6	78±5	80±4
Cardiac output l/min	5.2±0.7	3.8±0.3	4.8±0.4	4.6±0.6	3.4±0.3	3.5±0.4	3.9±0.6	4.2±0.4
	5.0±0.6	3.4±0.4	3.8±0.4	3.6±0.4	3.9±0.3	3.7±0.3	3.6±0.4	3.7±0.3
Heart rate beats/min	76±5	74±4	84±6	82±5	78±4	79±5	82±6	82±5
	78±6	72±3	74±3	76±4	76±5	74±4	76±4	76±4
Mean right atrial pressure mmHg	5±1	8±2	5±1	6±2	7±2	7±2	7±2	7±2
	7±1	7±1	6±1	6±1	7±2	8±2	8±2	8±2
Systemic vascular resistance dynes.sec.cm^{-5}	1430±124	1642±209	816±109	852±121	2047±242	2057±249	1579±156	1447±123
	1408±116	1764±164	989±94	922±97	1271±84	1513±106	1555±86	1556±79

Table 2. Plasma renin activity and plasma catecholamines before, during and after sodium nitroprusside infusion in ten (Group I) patients (first line in each panel) and in six (Group II) patients (second line in each panel) who were given intravenous propranolol (0.05 mg/kg) before nitroprusside infusion.

	Before Awake	Before Hypotension	30 min after hypotension	Before	Discontinuation of nitroprusside Minutes after			
					5	15	30	60
Plasma renin activity ng/ml/hr	1.25±0.2	2.09±0.3	4.52±1.1	4.81±1.24	5.26±1.38	4.23±1.14	2.21±0.6	1.74±0.6
	1.53±0.3	1.72±0.4	1.89±0.6	1.91±0.55	2.01±0.42	1.92±0.48	1.61±0.38	1.52±0.3
Norepinephrine Pg/ml	204±24	239±36	980±98	1102±121	1450±140	1320±112	450±49	280±22
	199±21	210±25	250±36	270±32	285±29	295±31	250±34	227±20
Epinephrine Pg/ml	52±13	58±27	190±44	230±39	280±41	250±33	120±26	99±14
	54±16	62±28	66±22	75±26	60±19	63±24	59±18	61±11
Dopamine Pg/ml	26±9	29±10	59±11	72±13	89±13	79±12	32±10	30±6
	21±8	25±7	29±8	32±7	28±6	26±6	24±4	27±6

Values are Mean ± SEM

Nitroprusside Dosage

The dose of nitroprusside utilized was significantly higher in Group 1 than in Group 2, despite comparable durations of hypotension in the two groups. Propranolol pretreatment decreased the dose of SNP by approximately 40 percent (from 4.3 to 2.6 μg/kg/min).

DISCUSSION

This study has three major findings. First, halothane-N_2O-O_2 anesthesia is associated with increased plasma renin activity. Second, nitroprusside-induced hypotension activates the sympatho-adrenal and renin-angiotensin systems. Third, propranolol pretreatment attenuates activation of these systems, decreases the dose of nitroprusside, and prevents rebound hypertension observed following withdrawal of nitroprusside. Before discussion of these results, an overview of the renin-angiotensin system is in order.

Renin is a glycoprotein enzyme (acid protease) formed by the juxtaglomerular cells (modified myoepithelium) in the walls of the afferent glomerular arteriole. Renin release is controlled by renal and extrarenal factors (Peach, 1977). There are two important renal influences. The first intrarenal influence is mechanical – any factor that tends to lower renal perfusion pressure elicits the secretion of renin, e.g. decreased systemic arterial pressure, decreased blood volume, or local vascular effects (renal arterial or aortic stenosis). The mechanism underlying these events is probably a decrease in tension within the wall of the glomerular afferent arterial vessel. The second intrarenal factor is ionic, i.e. reduction in sodium load to the kidney. This effect is probably mediated via the macula densa. Extrarenal influences include both neural and hormonal factors. The neural factor involves stimulation of the β_2-adrenergic receptors of the juxtaglomerular apparatus (inhibited by propranolol). Hormonal factors include angiotension II (inhibits renin release by a negative-feedback mechanism), ADH and circulating adrenal catecholamines stimulate secretion. Renin acts on angiotensinogen (renin substrate), an α-globulin, to yield the decapeptide angiotension I. This decapeptide has limited pharmacological activity, but it is cleaved by converting enzyme (peptidyl dipeptidase) to yield the highly active octapeptide, angiotensin II. This, in turn, undergoes hydrolysis by aminopeptidase to yield the heptapeptide angiotensin III, which is also pharmacologically active. Further cleavage yields peptides with little activity. Another recently described pathway involves the conversion of angiotensin I to des-Asp' angiotensin I, a nonapeptide. This is cleaved to the heptapeptide, angiotensin III, by the converting enzyme. Angiotensin II can increase the blood pressure by (1) vasoconstriction, which is mediated via (a) a direct action on vascular smooth muscle, (b) stimulation of the vasomotor center and (c) increased secretion of catecholamines; and (2) volume expansion by stimulation of aldosterone secretion, which leads to retention of sodium and water.

Nitrous oxide-halothane anesthesia produced hemodynamic effects similar to those described previously (Fahmy and Laver, 1976). A 12 percent decrease in mean arterial pressure was associated with a 75 percent increase in PRA in Group 1 patients. Such a significant rise in PRA was prevented with propranolol. An increase in PRA of 47 percent was reported by Khambata, Stone and Kman (1979).

Nitroprusside-induced hypotension was comparable in extent and duration in the two groups of patients. It was associated with increased activity of the sympatho-adrenal and renin-angiotensin systems in the untreated group. However, propranolol pretreatment attenuated the expected rise in the plasma catecholamines and PRA. These findings are in agreement with our previous report (Fahmy et al., 1979). Activation of the renin-angiotensin system has been demonstrated during vasodilator therapy in hypertensive patients (Kaneko et al., 1967) and during nitroprusside-induced hypotension in rats (Miller et al., 1977). Khambata et al. (1981) have used oral propranolol (180 mg) to attenuate renin release during nitroprusside-induced hypotension. It should be emphasized that intravenous propranolol is more predictable in its effects and can be repeated intraoperatively whenever it is required.

Propranolol pretreatment, in addition to attenuating catecholamine and renin release, prevented reflex tachycardia and decreased the dose of nitroprusside by 40 percent. Since cyanide release by SNP is dose-related, it is safe to conclude that a decreased amount of cyanide was present in the blood of Group 2 patients (Fahmy, 1981).

Rebound hypertension was observed following abrupt withdrawal of SNP in Group 1 but not in Group 2 patients, indicating that propranolol prevented such an event. Plasma catecholamines and PRA were elevated for at least 30 minutes in Group 1. Hemodynamically, systemic vascular resistance was significantly increased. These events were prevented by propranolol pretreatment. The results of this study can offer an explanation for the rebound hypertension. SNP administration results in two opposing factors (1) vasodilatation due to a direct action of the drug on vascular smooth muscle and (2) vasoconstriction which is produced by compensatory increases in PRA and plasma catecholamines. Because of the evanescent effects of SNP, its abrupt withdrawal leaves the vasoconstrictor forces unopposed. This leads to the hemodynamic events observed in Group 1 patients. These hemodynamic events can be catastrophic when SNP is discontinued in patients with congestive heart failure, myocardial infarction or following clipping of a cerebral aneurysm. Therefore, the use of propranolol prior to SNP withdrawal, should be considered in these situations.

Other methods suggested to prevent or attenuate rebound hypertension include slow withdrawal of SNP, combined use of hydralazine and propranolol, angiotensin II antagonists (e.g. intravenous saralasin), and converting enzyme inhibitors (e.g. teprotide and captopril). Intravenous saralasin has been demonstrated to prevent rebound hypertension following SNP withdrawal in rats (Delaney and Miller, 1980). However, the partial agonistic effect of this drug may preclude its use. It is important to note that the converting enzyme is also involved in the breakdown of bradykinin (the most powerful vasodilator known) and prostaglandins (Swartz et al., 1980). Thus, use of converting enzyme inhibitors not only inhibit the formation of angiotensin II, but also the breakdown of bradykinin and prostaglandins is inactivated.

In conclusion, this study has demonstrated that SNP infusion is associated with increased PRA and plasma catecholamines and that rebound hypertension follows the abrupt withdrawal of SNP. Pretreatment with intravenous propranolol decreases the dose of SNP, attenuates the release of catecholamines and renin into the circulation and prevents reflex tachycardia during the hypotensive phase, and prevents the occurrence of rebound hypertension upon discontinuation of SNP infusion.

Acknowledgements

The author is grateful to Professor Haralambos P. Gavras for his scientific advice and measurement of catecholamines and renin activity, to John T. Butler for his technical assistance and to Miss Ruth Anne Haneffant for her secretarial help.

REFERENCES

Delaney, T. J., and Miller, E. D., 1980, Rebound hypertension after sodium nitroprusside prevented by saralasin in rats, Anesthesiology, 52:154-156.

Fahmy, N. R., and Laver, M. B., 1976, Hemodynamic response to ganglionic blockade with pentolinium during N_2O-halothane anesthesia in man, Anesthesiology, 44:6-15.

Fahmy, N. R., Sunder, N., Moss, J., Slater, E., and Lappas, D. G., 1979, Tachyphylaxis to nitroprusside. Role of the renin-angiotensin system and catecholamines in its development, Anesthesiology, 51:S72.

Fahmy, N. R., 1981, Consumption of vitamin B_{12} during sodium nitroprusside administration in humans, Anesthesiology, 54:305-309.

Gerber, J. G., and Nies, A. S., 1979, Abrupt withdrawal of cardiovascular drugs, N.Engl.J.Med., 301:1234-1235.

Kaneko, Y., Ikeda, T., Takeda, T., and Ueda, H., 1967, Renin release
    during acute reduction of arterial pressure in normotensive
    subjects and in patients with renovascular hypertension,
    J.Clin.Invest., 46:705-716.
Khambatta, H. J., Stone, J. G., and Khan, E., 1979, Hypertension
    during anesthesia on discontinuation of sodium nitroprusside-
    induced hypotension, Anesthesiology, 51:127-130.
Khambatta, H. J., Stone, J. G., and Khan, E., 1981, Propranolol
    alters renin release during nitroprusside-induced hypotension
    and prevents hypertension on discontinuation of nitroprusside,
    Anesth.Analg., 60:569-573.
Miller, E. D., Ackerly, J. A., Vaughan, D., Jr., Peach, M. J., and
    Epstein, R. M., 1977, The renin-angiotensin system during
    controlled hypotension with sodium nitroprusside, Anes-
    thesiology, 47:257-262.
Packer, M., Meller, J., Medina, N., Gorlin, R., and Herman, M. V.,
    1979, Rebound hemodynamic events after the abrupt withdrawal
    of nitroprusside in patients with severe chronic heart fail-
    ure, N.Engl.J.Med., 301:1193-1197.
Peach, M. J., 1977, Renin-angiotensin system, Physiol Rev.,
    57:313-370.
Peuler, J. D., and Johnson, G. A., 1977, Simultaneous single isotope
    radioenzymatic assay of plasma norepinephrine, epinephrine and
    dopamine, Life Sci., 21:625-636.
Sealey, J. E., Gerten-Banes, J., and Laragh, J. H., 1972, The renin
    system: variations measured by radioimmunoassay or bioassay,
    Kidney Int., 1:240-253.
Swartz, S. L., Williams, G. H., Hollenberg, N. K., Levine, L., Dluhy,
    R. G., and Moore, T. J., 1980, Captopril-induced changes in
    prostaglandin production; Relationship to vascular responses
    in normal man, J.Clin.Invest., 65:1257-1264.

IS THERE STILL ANY INDICATION FOR APPLICATION OF VOLATILE

ANESTHETICS DURING INDUCTION OF HYPOTENSION IN NEUROSURGERY?

G. Cunitz

Department of Anesthesiology and Intensive Care
University of Bochum
Knappschafts-Krankenhaus

    Deliberately induced hypotension is quite a useful and wide-spread technique in neuroanesthesia. It is widely used in the surgical treatment of arterial aneurysms and arteriovenous mal-formations, sometimes also in cases of meningeoms or other vascular-ized tumors. The decision to use induced hypotension is a surgical one, the degree of hypotension should be agreed on jointly by the neurosurgeon and anesthetist, each putting forward his arguments. The importance of induced hypotension is well documented: diminished blood loss and reduced brain swelling and intracranial pressure in the presence of impaired autoregulation. Hypotension is the method of preference in aneurysm surgery. It's influence on the incidence of rupture, however, is not as well established as one might expect from the wide application of this technique. Reports on the cor-relation between systemic arterial pressure and the incidence of rupture of an aneurysm are somewhat conflicting (Gordon 1975). Some other factors such as configuration of the aneurysm sack, condition of the cerebral arteries and time of foregoing bleeding also seem to be involved. Very often it is not the aneurysm itself that ruptures but a surrounding vessel. The neurosurgeon expects that hypotension produces a somewhat softer aneurysmal sack, and that the blood ves-sels in the vicinity of the aneurysm are less tortuous. The dis-cussion about the adequate level of hypotension also contributes to this uncertainty: some hospitals use very low limits, e.g. 65 mm Hg systolic pressure or less (Hunter, 1975; Niedermeyer, 1977), other hospitals work quite successfully with higher pressure limits. We lower BP only in a moderate way: at the moment of clipping the aneurysm or wrapping it in a piece of muscle BP is held at about 80 mm Hg systolic pressure (a mean of 60). The safe individual level, however, is chosen during the surgical procedure and depends on well-known factors such as the state of the cardiovascular system, location of the aneurysm and cerebral perfusion.

For many years halothane was the standard anesthetic in neuro-surgical procedures. When, however, the application of i.v. anal-gesics and sedatives became more and more widespread in general anesthesia, halothane lost its predominant position in neuro-anesthesia as well. Today neuroleptanalgesia (NLA), eventually completed by a barbiturate i.v. drip, is regarded as the principal technique of anesthesia for intracranial surgical interventions. Some disadvantageous effects of halothane were detected, as was the case with enflurane which was introduced later. NLA or i.v. anes-thetics gave better results:

1. Intracranial pressure (ICP) clearly increases after halothane, predominantly due to augmentation of cerebral blood volume (McDowall et al., 1968; Jennett et al., 1979) and to a small degree due to real increase of the brain tissue itself as Dr. Schettini (1980) pointed out. Enflurane also elevates ICP, but to a lesser extent (Cunitz et al., 1976).

2. Cerebral blood flow increases. Luxury perfusion is established which does not seem to produce better conditions for the patient than when other agents are given.

3. Halothane and enflurane are followed by myocardial depression - dependent on respective MAC values, whereas neuroleptanalgesia, in its usual dosage, is not. Both techniques cause a peripheral vasodilation, which is more pronounced in NLA. Blood pressure falls after halothane and enflurane. It may fall in the course of neuroleptanalgesia.

4. Cerebral perfusion pressure (CPP = BP-ICP) is reduced to a greater extent by inhalation anesthetics than by NLA. CPP is lowered by a BP decrease or an ICP increase. Its lower limit is about 50 mm Hg (Zwetnow, 1968). In neuroanesthesia, there may occasionally be reason to combine NLA and inhalation anesthesia. One of the more important reasons for this practice is to cut off arterial pressure peaks during anesthesia and operation. Slow or sudden pressure elevations may occur, e.g. when the patient is in the sitting position or when the brain stem is irritated. In this situation it is useful to give the patient an additional volume of halothane or enflurane (0.7 and 1% respectively). In this way, BP is well controlled.

Now an example (Figure 1):

A 63 year-old woman suffering from a syringomyelia is admin-istered a sequence of enflurane (1.5%), methoxyflurane and halothane (1%), halothane and enflurane in nearly equivalent concentrations. Basic anesthesia is provided by NLA. Besides the different ICP-increasing effects of the applied anesthetics, it can be clearly seen that blood pressure falls remarkably in all three situations, and comes back to its initial level when the anesthetics are switched off.

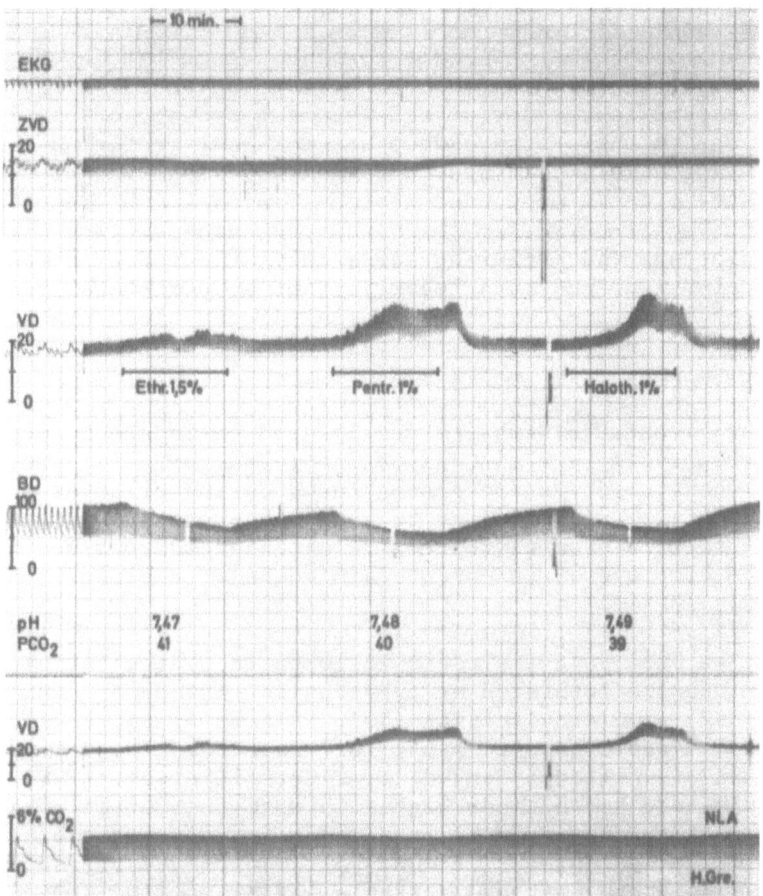

Fig. 1.   Effects of enflurane (Ethr.), methoxyflurane (Pentr.) and
          halothane on centralvenous pressure (ZVD), intracranial
          pressure (VD) and blood pressure (BD). Basic anesthesia is
          a neuroleptanalgesia. ICP (intracranial pressure) was
          measured via a ventricular catheter.

     Thus we have seen that halothane or enflurane are of value in
antihypertensive therapy during anesthesia.

     Halothane and enflurane are also of value when induced hypo-
tension for intracranial surgery is desired. There are some reasons
to justify this conclusion: the blood pressure-lowering effect of
both agents is safe when they are applied in addition to basic
anesthesia. Sudden pressure drops do not occur. Critical cardiovascular situations do not arise, provided concentrations are not too
high, i.e. not more than 1 MAC halothane or enflurane. In general,
halothane and enflurane produce comparable negative effects on heart

muscle contractility. When applied in equianesthetic concentrations
in animal models, enflurane seems to have a somewhat lesser effect
than halothane, as Fischer (1976) and Siepmann et al. (1976) pointed
out. The effect on the peripheral vascular system, of halothane and
enflurane due to the pressure drop are somewhat confusing and controversial. In general, both agents diminish peripheral vascular resistance. These effects are counteracted - in part - by regulatory
mechanisms (Dudziak, 1980). The blood pressure-lowering properties
of both halothane and enflurane are mainly effected by direct myocardial depression, and to a lesser extent by peripheral vasodilation. In clinical practice, enflurane lowers blood pressure to a
greater degree, and more quickly, than halothane when given in equianesthetic volumes.

Of the vasoactive drugs currently used to induce hypotension,
sodium nitroprusside and nitroglycerine reveal arterial pressure
overshoot when the drugs are discontinued during or after intracranial surgery. This may lead to very dangerous situations:
especially after sodium nitroprusside blood pressure rises to levels
at which development of cerebral brain edema or rebleeding must be
considered.

Today we know that the renin-angiotensin system and circulating
catecholamines are activated by hypotension induced by sodium nitroprusside (SNP) or nitroglycerine (NG). Plasma renin, angiotensin II
and catecholamines are responsible for the rebound hypertension. The
effect of SNP is well documented, e.g. Cotrell et al. (1980) found
plasma renin levels 3.8 times higher than at the outset of application. Trimetaphane - rarely used in anesthesia today - also shows
slight endocrinological activation. Blood pressure overshoot does
not occur. Among the methods suitable for overcoming these negative
side effects, β-blocking agents (propranolol) are of value (Khambatta
and Stone, 1981; Fahmy, 1981). We use 3 x 80 mg propranolol per os
beginning the day before operation. Halothane and enflurane, however, are also suited to neuralizing or diminishing the endocrinological activity. Miyazaki and coworkers (1980) recommend halothane
when sodium nitroprusside or nitroglycerine are used for hypotension.
According to their studies the endocrinological consequences can be
significantly mitigated in this manner. Halothane and enflurane are
well proven depressors of sympathetic nervous system activity.

We now turn to a few examples of the influence of antihypertensive drugs on BP and ICP. The latter point has to be taken into
consideration when a drug is used in neuroanesthesia. From many
investigators mentioned here - pars to toto Dr. Turner and coworkers
(1977) - we know that sodium nitroprusside increases intracranial
pressure by augmenting cerebral blood volume. As Dr. Pickerodt
(1981) stated during this symposium nitroglycerine has a minor
increasing effect as well.

Now to some examples:

1. A 28-year-old male patient (70 kg b.w.) with a frontal lobe
    traumatic lesion received sodium nitroprusside (200 µg) within
    3 minutes. Blood pressure dropped and ICP dropped too. I
    suppose that in this case a decrease in ICP occurred because
    cerebral autoregulation had broken down. ICP follows BP
    passively (Figure 2).
2. The same patient as in Figure 2 was injected with 270 mg
    diazoxide (Hypertonalum®), which we often use to neutralize a
    sudden blood pressure increase during or after anesthesia in
    neurosurgery: blood pressure falls moderately and ICP decreases
    as well (Figure 3).
3. The same patient receives 0.2 mg pindolol (Visken®), a
    β-blocking agent. BP and ICP drop together (Figure 4).
4. The same patient is now administered urapidil (Ebrantil®), a new
    antihypertensive drug, the mode of action of which is based on
    peripheral vasodilation. BP falls after infusion of 1, 2 oder
    3 mg per minute. Upper limit of intracranial pressure increases
    slightly. Arterial pulsations within the increase, is often a
    sign of reduced cerebral compliance (Figure 5).
5. A 69-year-old male patient, suffering from severe head injury,
    shows extremely high ICP values. He is administered mannitol
    (40 g) and furosemide (20 mg) without effect. But ICP and even
    BP are rising instead of falling. The injection of 25 mg hydra-
    lazine (Nepresol®), however, strikingly lowers ICP as well as BP
    (Figure 6).

The above-mentioned antihypertensive drugs are also suited to
lowering blood pressure during anesthesia and operation. And they
are often used. Their effect on intracranial pressure and cerebral
blood flow, however, must be kept in mind when they are injected.

Since the first studies of Dr. McDowall it is well known that
SNP presents a problem of cynanide toxicity if administered too
rapidly over time or in an ultimately too high dosage in patients who
seem resistant to its hypotensive effect. NG is less dangerous with
regard to toxicity, but methemoglobinemia may occur. Use of halothane or enflurane can reduce the doses of SNP and NG needed to
achieve the low blood pressure aimed for by the anesthetist. Three
reasons for using enflurane or halothane in deliberately induced
hypotension should be pointed out:

1. Safe and smooth induction
2. Neutralization of endocrinological reactions
3. Reduction of doses of SNP and NG.

A fourth reason is more speculative: avoidance of postoperative
vasospasm. The occurrence of a vasospasm, sometimes locally, sometimes generalized, is a major problem after aneurysmal surgery.
There have been many attempts to avoid this complication which often

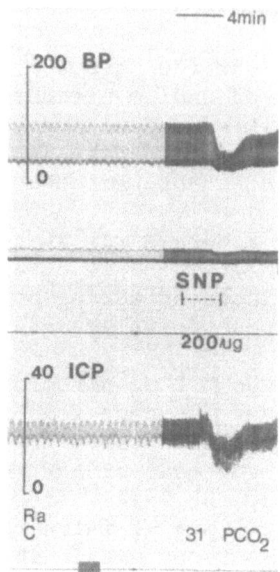

Fig. 2.   Effect of sodium nitroprusside (SNP) on blood pressure (BP)
          and intracranial pressure (ICP). The patient is suffering
          from head injury (Glasgow Coma Scale 5). ICP was measured
          by an epidural Gaeltec Transducer.

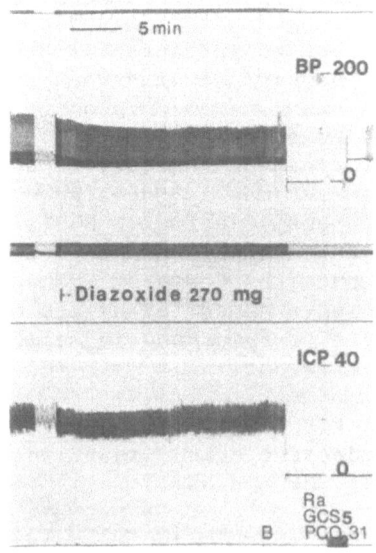

Fig. 3.   Effect of diazoxide. The same patient as in Figure 2.

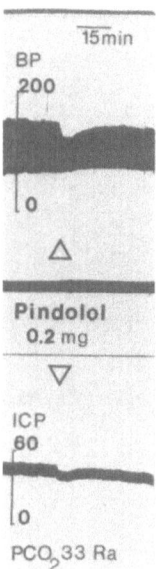

Fig. 4.   Effect of pindolol.   The same patient as in Figure 2 and 3.

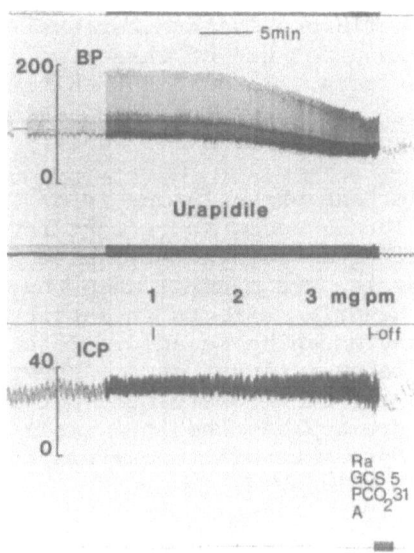

Fig. 5.   Effect of urapidile, a new antihypertensive drug.   The same
         patient as in Figure 2-4.

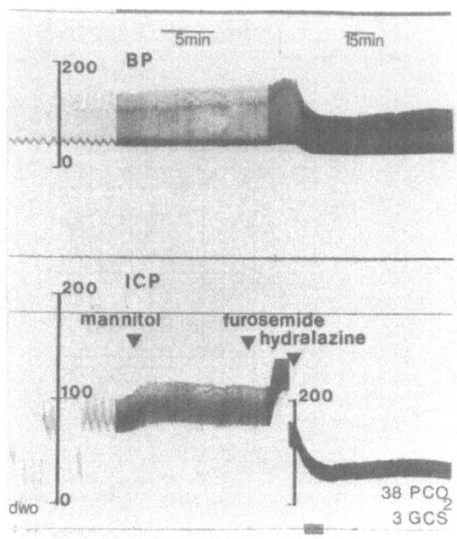

Fig. 6.   Application of mannitol, furosemide and hydralazine in case
          of an extremely high ICP. The patient is flaccid (Glasgow
          Coma Scale 3).

leads to death or permanent neurological deficits: application of
phenoxybenzamine, papaverine, dopamine, serotonin antagonists and
others. Their effects, however, often remain uncertain. Halothane,
and to a lesser degree enflurane, dilate cerebral vessels. This
appears to be a good reason for use of these two inhalation anesthetics in aneurysmal surgery. They do not initiate vasoconstriction
that might end in a vasospasm. For the same reason we avoid hyperventilation during intracerebral vascular surgery.

    Application of halothane or enflurane is of value for inducing
hypotension whereby enflurane seems to be more favorable. The blood
pressure-lowering effects are satisfactory; side effects with regard
to the cardiovascular system are minimal when the dosage is restricted to 1 MAC. The negative effects on intracranial pressure and
cerebral perfusion pressure can be managed. Both agents are administered as supplements to basic anesthesia - generally neuroleptanalgesia (NLA). In this way their doses need not be dangerously high.
Enflurane or halothane are applied when the skull has already been
opened so that no major pressure will occur despite a potential
slight increase in brain volume.

    These measures permit adequate lowering and maintenance of blood
pressure at a safe level. Nitroprusside or nitroglycerine may be
administered additionally. In some cases, the blood pressure-
lowering effects of enflurane and halothane readily suffice to complete the operation.

REFERENCES

Cottrell, J. E., Gupta, B., and Turndorf, H., 1980, Induced hypo-
    tension, in: "Anesthesia and Neurosurgery," J. E. Cottrell and
    H. Turndorf, eds., The C.V. Mosby Company, St. Louis - Toronto
    - London, pp.387-400.
Cunitz, G., Danhauser, I., and Bruß, P., 1976, Die Wirkung von
    Enflurane (Ethrane®) im Vergleich zu Halothan auf den intra-
    craniellen Druck, Anaesthesist, 25:323-330.
Dudziak, R., 1980, Lehrbuch der Anaesthesiologie, F.K. Schattauer
    Verlag, Stuttgart - New York.
Fahmy, N. R., 1981, Rebound hypertension following controlled hypo-
    tension: Aetiology and treatment, during this sympsosium.
Fisher, K. J., 1976, Tierexperimentelle Untersuchungen zur Quanti-
    fizierung der direkten Myocardeffekte äquinarkotischer
    Ethrane- und Halothan- Konzentrationen, in: "Inhalations-
    anaesthesie mit Ethrane," J. B. Brückner, ed., Springer
    Verlag, Berlin - Heidelberg - New York, Anaesthesiology and
    Recuscitation, Vol.99, p.43-62.
Gordon, E., 1975, Induced hypotension and hypothermia, in: "A Basis
    and Practice of Neuroanaesthesia," E. Gordon, ed., Excerpta
    Medica, Amsterdam - Oxford - New York, 219-238.
Hunter, A. R., 1975, Neurosurgical anaesthesia, Blackwell Scientific
    Publications, Oxford - London - Edinburgh - Melbourne.
Jennett, W. B., Barker, J., Fitch, W., and McDowall, D. G., 1969,
    Effects of anaesthesia on intracranial pressure in patients
    with space-occupying lesions, Lancet II, 61.
Khambatta, H. J., and Stone, J. G., 1981, Effect of propranolol on
    plasma renin-angiotensin system and catecholamines duri:.
    nitroprusside induced hypotension, Br.J.Anaesth., 53:306.
McDowall, D. G., Jennett, W. B., and Barker, J., 1968, The effects
    of halothane and trichloroethylene on cerebral perfusion and
    metabolism and on intracranial pressure, in: "Progress in
    Brain Research,", Vol.30, cerebral circulation, W. Luyendijk,
    ed., Elsevier, p.83-86.
Miyazaki, M., Mitsufuji, T., and Yukioka, K., 1980, Endocrine
    responses in hypotensive anaesthesia, 7th World Congress of
    Anaesthesiologists, Hamburg.
Niedermeier, B., 1977, Die kontrollierte Hypotension bei der
    Operation intrakranieller Gefäßmißbildungen, Anaesthesiologie
    und Intensivmedizin, 18, 32 pp.72-77.
Pickerodt, V. W. A., 1981, Recent aspects of hypotensive drug effects
    on intracranial pressure, during this symposium.
Schettini, A., 1980, Incompatibility of halogenated anesthetics with
    brain surgery, in: "Intracranial Pressure IV," K. Shulman, A.
    Marmarou, J. D. Miller, D. P. Becker, G. M. Hochwald, and M.
    Brock, eds., Springer Verlag Berlin - Heidelberg - New York,
    p.599-602.
Siepmann, H., Lennartz, H., und Pütz, E., 1976, Die dosisabhängige
    Beeinflussung der Kontraktilität des isolierten

Papillarmuskels der Katze durch Enflurane und Halothane, in:
"Inhalationsanaesthesie mit Ethrane," J. B. Brückner, ed.,
Springer Verlag Berlin - Heidelberg - New York, Anaesthes-
iology and Resuscitation, Vol.99, p.71-81.

Turner, J.M., Powell, D., Gibson, R. M., and McDowall, D. G., 1977,
Intracranial pressure changes in neurosurgical patients during
hypotension induced with sodium nitroprusside or trimetaphan,
Brit.J.Anaesth., 49:419-425.

Zwetnow, N., Kjällquist, A., and Siesjö, B. K., 1968, Cerebral blood
flow during intracranial hypertension related to tissue
hypoxia and to acidosis in cerebral extracellular fluids, in:
"Progress in Brain Research," Vol.30, cerebral circulation, W.
Luyendijk, ed., Elsevier, Amsterdam - London - New York,
p.87-92.

INTERACTIONS OF ANESTHETIC DRUGS AND MUSCLE RELAXANTS

WITH THOSE DRUGS COMMONLY USED FOR CONTROLLED HYPOTENSION

V. Hempel and F. Münch

Department of Anesthesia
University of Tubingen
Calwestr. 7, 7400 Tubingen-1, FRG

In general anesthesia, potent drugs are often used concomitantly. The simultaneous application of two or more drugs may lead to unexpected effects, which can be ascribed to interactions (i.e., in vivo interferences) or to incompatibilities which occur in vitro when drugs are mixed together, the latter being a pharmaceutical problem.

This review deals with drug interactions associated with controlled hypotension in anesthesia. The hypotensive agents which are taken into consideration are the nitro compounds sodium nitroprusside and nitroglycerine and the ganglioplegic agent trimetaphan. Whereas the practical importance of trimetaphan has decreased, with respect to drug interactions it is the more interesting hypotensive agent.

Two groups of drug interactions can be distinguished. One involves pharmacokinetic interactions. This means, that one drug modifies the distribution, the metabolism or the excretion of the other one, thus leading to an increase or a prolongation of its clinical effect - for example, the prolongation of ketamine effects under halothane anesthesia by inhibition of ketamine biodegradation (White et al., 1975). The second group involves pharmacodynamic interactions, that is, a modification of an effect or side effect by action at the same receptor site or at different receptor sites which trigger one effect, an example of which is the enhancement of muscle relaxation by inhalation anesthetics such as halogenated ether compounds (Wand, 1979).

The manufacturers' notices about side effects and drug interactions of the hypotensive agents under consideration only provide basic information. It is warned not to employ other antihypertensive agents concomitantly, which seems to be something between a banality and an overstatement. Interactions with anesthetics and muscle relaxants are not reported. This may reflect lack of knowledge or concern about these interferences. But many interactions between the drugs under consideration seem to be possible, but have not yet been investigated to date, and some have been investigated and should be known.

PHARMACOKINETIC INTERACTIONS

Plasma Protein Binding

This can result in enhancement of drug effects, when one drug is displaced from the binding protein by another one, thus increasing the free concentration of the first one. The prerequisite for the potential of displacing other drugs from protein binding are a plasma protein binding of more than 90% and a high absolute dosage (Remmer, 1974). This does not at all apply to the nitro compounds. The plasma protein binding of nitroglycerine is estimated to be about 60%, and sodium nitroprusside is rapidly broken down in the erythrocytes and does not bind to plasma proteins to a significant amount. Both hypotensive agents are employed in very small doses. The plasma protein binding of trimetaphan is higher than that of the nitro compounds (less than 90%), but is also unlikely to interfere with plasma protein binding of other drugs. It is, however, bound by the cholinesterases, the activity of which is thereby inhibited significantly, as shown by the experiments of Sklar and Lanks (1977). The inhibition of the serum cholinesterase activity by trimetaphan is of the noncompetitive type. This explains Tewfik's observation of prolonged apnea in patients treated with trimetaphan and succinylcholine (Tewfik, 1957). It is conceivable that the effect of propanidid (Doenicke et al., 1968; Ellis, 1968) is also prolonged by trimetaphan. The concomitant use of propanidid and trimetaphan, however, is unusual, and the practice of succinylcholine drip for continuous muscle relaxation has largely been abandoned.

It remains unclear whether trimetaphan is broken down by human serum cholinesterase to a significant amount. Gertner (1955) has demonstrated that only 30-40% of the unchanged drug is excreted by the renal route. It may be, that hepatic esterases play the main role in trimetaphan inactivation.

Sklar and Lanks (1977) have also shown that sodium nitroprusside has no effect on the serum cholinesterase activity. It is unlikely that nitroglycerine affects this group of enzymes.

Renal Excretion

Animal experiments (Wang, 1977) suggest that renal perfusion is more likely to be impaired by trimetaphan hypotension than by nitro-

prusside. In man, renal perfusion remains unaffected by nitroprusside when it is used for afterload-reduction in cardiac patients
(Meseda et al., 1981). Renal excretion is the main mechanism of
muscle relaxant elimination. Thus, deep trimetaphan-induced hypotension may lead to prolonged muscle relaxation due to impaired
excretion. There is, however, evidence that the prolonged effect of
curare type muscle relaxants is due to an interaction at the receptor
site (see below).

Organ Perfusion

The commonly used hypotensive drugs do not change the distribution of organ perfusion to a significant amount (Bergmann et al.,
1980); Wang, 1977), but they are able to abolish the hemodynamic
changes associated with hypovolemia. The clinical observation that
patients with low cardiac output need only small doses of drugs
acting on the central nervous system can be explained as follows:
whereas the non-vital organs are less perfused than normal, cerebral
perfusion remains constant, and so a greater portion of the given
dose reaches its site of action in the brain. Controlled hypotension
restores the distribution of organ perfusion between the brain and
the other organs, with the result that now a normal dose is required.
This should apply to all drugs the effect of which is limited by
tissue distribution rather than biodegradation or renal excretion,
for example fentanyl (Stoeckel et al., 1979).

As a matter of changed organ perfusion, the prolonged pancuronium effect under nitroglycerine hypotension has been discussed by
Glisson et al. (1980). The authors raised the hypothesis that this
interaction could be due to a greater deposition of muscle relaxant
at the site of action resulting from an improved muscle perfusion.
In this case, the same prolongation of relaxation should be seen with
other relaxants than pancuronium, which is not the case, and with
sodium nitroprusside as a hypotensive agent, which also could not be
demonstrated.

PHARMACODYNAMIC INTERACTIONS

Detoxification of Nitroprusside/Vitamin B_{12}

Since the work of Amess et al., we know that prolonged application of nitrous oxide results in vitamin B_{12} depletion (Nunn and
Chanarin, 1978). A vitamin B_{12} depletion has also not unexpectedly
been found after nitroprusside hypotension (Fahmy, 1981). Thus, an
interaction of nitrous oxide and nitroprusside would be conceivable.
The cyanide inactivation by binding to vitamin B_{12}, however, is the
less important detoxification mechanism (Tinker and Michenfelder,
1976), whereas the more important thiocyanate formation by the enzyme

rhodanese is not impaired by nitrous oxide. This more important
pathway can be enhanced by the concomitant application of thiosulphate as recommended by Schulz et al. (1979). It would be of
interest to see whether the decrease of vitamin B_{12} levels during
sodium nitroprusside application can be prevented by the concomitant
infusion of thiosulphate.

Pharmacodynamic Interactions Affecting Hemodynamics

Since all potent inhalation anesthetics decrease cardiac output,
the combination of inhalation anesthesia and controlled hypotension
makes it easier to achieve the desired level of blood pressure than
is the case when controlled hypotension is performed under neurolept
anesthesia. Wildsmith and coworkers (Wildsmith et al., 1973), however, found that nitroprusside hypotension during halothane anesthesia in spontaneously breathing patients resulted in increased
cardiac output.

During controlled hypotension with the nitro compounds, a rise
of heart rate due to sympathetic stimulation is a normal finding.
This effect seems to be more pronounced under neurolept anesthesia,
requiring beta blockers. With respect to heart rate, the combination
of the nitro compounds and halothane with its accompanying bradycardia is the better choice than neuroleptanesthesia/nitro compounds.

Interactions on Pulmonary Gas Exchange

Wildsmith et al. (1975) were the first to report on blood gas
changes under nitroprusside-induced hypotension.

These findings can be explained by the suppression of hypoxic
vascular response (Von Euler and Liljestrand, 1946; West, 1977) by
sodium nitroprusside (Hilt et al., 1979). The effect of nitroglycerine on this protective mechanism against shunting seems to be
less marked (Colley et al., 1979). There are controversial reports
on the effect of potent inhalation anesthetics on the pulmonary
hypoxic vascular response (Sykes et al., 1978). The anesthetist
should, however, keep in mind that the combination of inhalation
anesthesia and controlled hypotension using sodium nitroprusside may
have an additive effect on pulmonary shunting.

Pharmacodynamic Interactions of Muscle Relaxants and Hypotensive Agents

The pharmacodynamic interactions of muscle relaxants and ganglioplegic agents have been investigated by Deacock and Davies (1958).
It is conceivable that agents affecting acetylcholine receptors in

the sympathetic ganglia have the same effect on the acetylcholine
receptors of the motor end plate when administered in sufficient
doses. In reverse fashion, it is well known, that muscle relaxants
of the curare type can exert a ganglioplegic effect. The experiments
of Deacock and Davies performed on a rat diaphragm suggest that the
neuromuscular blocking effect of trimetaphan is of the curare type
(Deacock and Davies, 1958). Fade during tetanic stimulation was
observed; yet in contrast to other ganglioplegics, the effect of
trimetaphan was not reversed by neostigmine but instead enhanced.
The authors postulate that this neuromuscular blocking effect of
trimetaphan may prolong the effect of muscle relaxants of the curare
type significantly under clinical conditions. Such an interaction
may be noticed by anesthetists working routinely with nerve stimul-
ators to monitor muscle relaxant effects.

As mentioned above, Glisson et al. (1980) have demonstrated that
nitroglycerine enhanced the muscle relaxation achieved with pancuronium, but not with other muscle relaxants. The elimination of pancuronium from serum is not affected. Other vasodilator drugs have no
effect on the pancuronium block. The mechanism of this interaction
is not yet understood. The prolonged block has the properties of a
normal curare type block and is reversed by neostigmine. It is
likely to be an interaction at the receptor site. Perhaps, nitroglycerine alters the affinity of these receptors to pancuronium.

REFERENCES

Bergman, S., Hoffman, W. E., Jozefiak, A., Miletich, D. J., Gan,
        B. J., and Albrecht, R. F., 1980, Regional hemodynamic changes
        of sodium nitroprusside vs. nitroglycerin, Anesthesiology,
        53:S 79.
Colley, P. S., Cheney, F. W., and Hlastala, M. P., 1979, Ventilation-
        perfusion effects of nitroglycerin, Anesthesiology, 51:S 372.
Deacock, A. R. C., and Davies, T. D. W., 1958, The influence of cer-
        tain ganglionic blocking agents on neuromuscular transmission,
        Birt.J.Anaesth., 30:217-225.
Doenicke, A., Krumey, I., Kugler, J., and Klempa, J., 1968, Experi-
        mental studies of the breakdown of epontol, Brit.J.Anaesth.,
        40:415-429.
Ellis, F. R., 1968, The neuromuscular interaction of propanidid with
        suxamethonium and tubocurarine, Brit.J.Anaesth., 40:818-824.
Fahmy, N. R., 1981, Consumption of vitamin B_{12} during sodium nitro-
        prusside administration in humans, Anesthesiology, 54:305-309.
Gertner, S. B., Little, D. M., and Bonnycastle, D. D., 1955, Urinary
        excretion of arfonad by patients undergoing "controlled hypo-
        tension" during surgery, Anesthesiology, 16:495-502.
Glisson, S. N., Sanchez, M. M., El-Etr, A. A., and Lim, R. A., 1980,
        Niroglycerin and the neuromuscular blockade produced by
        gallamine, succinylcholine, d-tubocurarine, and pancuronium,
        Anesth.Analg., 59:117-122.

Hill, A. B., Sykes, M. K., and Reynes, A., 1979, A hypoxic pulmonary
    vasoconstrictor response in dogs during and after infusion of
    sodium nitroprusside, Anesthesiology, 50:484-488.
Nunn, J. F., and Chanarin, I., 1978, Nitrous oxide and vitamin B_{12},
    Editorial.Brit.J.Anaesth., 50:1089-1090.
Maseda, J., Hilberman, M., Derby, G. C., Spencer, R. J., Stinson,
    E. B., and Myers, B. D., 1981, The renal effects of sodium
    nitroprusside in postoperative cardiac surgical patients,
    Anesthesiology, 54:284-288.
Remmer, H., 1974, Wirkungsveränderungen von Arzneimitteln durch
    gegenseitige Störung ihrer Eiweißbindung und ihres Abbaus,
    Dtsch.med.Wochenschr., 99:413-423.
Schulz, V., Bonn, R., Kämmerer, H., Kriegel, R., and Ecker, N., 1979,
    Counteraction of cyanide poisoning by thiosulphate when
    administering sodium nitroprusside as a hypotensive treatment,
    Klin.Wochenschr., 57:905-907.
Sklar, G. S., and Lanks, K. W., 1977, Effects of trimetaphan and
    sodium nitroprusside on hydrolysis of succinylcholine in
    vitro, Anesthesiology, 47:31-33.
Stoeckel, H., Hengstmann, J. H., and Schüttler, J., 1979, Pharmaco-
    kinetics of fentanyl as a possible explanation for recurrence
    of respiratory depression, Brit.J.Anaesth., 51:741-745.
Sykes, M. K., Gibbs, J. M., Loh, L., Marin, J. B. L., Obdrzalek, J.,
    and Arnot, R. N., 1978, Preservation of the pulmonary vaso-
    constrictor response to alveolar hypoxia during the admin-
    istration of halothane to dogs, Brit.J.Anaesth., 50:1185-1196.
Tewfik, G. I., 1957, Trimetaphan - its effect on the pseudocholin-
    esterase level of man, Anaesthesia, 12:326-329.
Tinker, J. H., and Michenfelder, J. D., 1976, Sodium nitroprusside:
    Pharmacology, toxicology and therapeutics, Anesthesiology,
    45:340-354.
Von Euler, U. S., and Liljestrand, G., 1946, Observations on the
    pulmonary arterial blood pressure in the cat, Acta Physiol.
    Scand., 12:301-322.
Wang, H. H., Liu, L. M. P., and Katz, R. L., 1977, A comparison of
    the cardiovascular effects of sodium nitroprusside and
    trimetaphan, Anesthesiology, 46:40-48.
Waud, B. E., 1979, Decrease of dose requirement of d-tubocurarine by
    volatile anesthetics, Anesthesiology, 51:298-302.
West, J. B., 1977, Regional differences in the lung, Academic Press
    London.
White, P. F., Johnston, R. R., and Pudwill, C. R., 1975, Interaction
    of ketamine and halothane in rats, Anesthesiology, 42:179-186.
Wildsmith, J. A. W., Drummond, G. B., and MacRea, W. R., 1975, Blood-
    gas changes during induced hypotension with sodium nitroprus-
    side, Brit.J.Anaesth., 47:1205-1210.
Wildsmith, J. A., Marshall, R. L., Jenkinson, J. L., MacRae, W. R.,
    and Scott, D. B., 1973, Haemodynamic effects of sodium nitro-
    prusside during nitrous oxide/halothane anaesthesia, Brit.J.
    Anaesth., 45:71-74.

II

CEREBRAL BLOOD FLOW AND METABOLISM UNDER
CONDITIONS OF SYSTEMIC HYPOTENSION

DIRECT AND INDIRECT CEREBRAL EFFECTS

OF DELIBERATE HYPOTENSION

J. E. Cottrell

SUNY Downstate School of Medicine
Brooklyn, New York
USA

The benefits of inducing hypotension during anesthesia and surgery were first described by Harvey Cushing in 1917. However, laboratory investigations did not begin until 1944 when Phemister demonstrated increased survival of rabbits after hypotension was induced with hemorrhage when compared with neurogenic blockade. In 1946 Gardner removed 1600 ml of blood from the dorsalis pedis artery thereby reducing systolic blood pressure from 140 to 100 torr. In 1948 Gillies used subarachnoid block to reduce blood pressure and stated that "a low head of arterial pressure associated with vaso-dilation and a normal blood volume carried less potential danger than the illusory higher pressure which accompanies vasoconstriction and a reduced blood volume". The use and development of methonium compounds for ganglionic blockade occurred from 1948 to 1951. These drugs were recommended to treat hypertension and to afford a hypotensive state during operation that would significantly reduce bleeding from the operative field. In 1953 Boyan reduced blood pressure to a mean of 50 torr with hexamethonium bromide in a group of patients undergoing radical cancer surgery. Surgery was facilitated, blood loss was reduced, and adverse effects were not observed. The popularity of this technique has varied but today finds wide acceptance especially during microvascular surgery.

METHODS TO INDUCE HYPOTENSION

Blood pressure is decreased chemically by direct arterial or venous dilators or by ganglionic blocking drugs. Perfusion pressure decreases proportionate to the decrease in vascular flow resistance, and within wide limits adequate tissue blood flow persists. Fine pressure adjustments which may be needed to achieve the desired level

49

of hypotension can be obtained by superimposing changes in body
position, altering airway pressure, controlling heart rate or the
addition of other vasoactive drugs whose effects may compliment the
primary hypotensive drug. A safe hypotensive technique should be
easy to control, not alter vital organ blood flow, have a short
plasma and biological half-life, be nontoxic, produce no toxic
metabolites, or produce other untoward physiologic responses.

COMMONLY USED DRUGS

Sodium Nitroprusside (SNP) is most widely used to induce hypotension because of its short half-life, and maintenance of vital
organ blood flow and oxygen supply even at perfusion pressures of
40 torr. Sodium nitroprusside primarily dilates resistance vessels
either by interfering with sulfhydryl groups or intracellular activation of calcium. Cardiac output and cerebral blood flow (CBF) are
unaffected by SNP at a mean arterial pressure (MAP) of 40-50 torr.

Adverse effects occur after SNP and include cyanide (CN) and
thiocyanate (TCN) toxicity, rebound hypertension (RH), intracranial
hypertension, blood coagulation abnormalities, and hypothyroidism
(Table 1).

Cyanide is produced when SNP is metabolized. One mg of SNP
contains 0.44 mg of CN. Toxic blood levels (greater than 100 µg%)
occur when greater than 1 mg/kg SNP is administered within 2½ hours
or when greater than 0.5 mg/kg is administered within 24 hours.
Death from CN has been reported after 4-12 mg/kg CN. Death following SNP secondary to CN has been reported when blood CN level was
400 µg%. Greater risk of CN toxicity exists in those patients
nutritionally deficient in the cobalamins (vitamin B_{12} compounds) or
in dietary substances containing specific sulfur donors. Monitoring
of blood CN and pH will detect abnormalities in those patients at
risk and in whom larger amounts than those previously recommended are
used. Treatment should consist of intraveous (IV) thiosulfate except
in those patients with abnormal renal function. Hydroxocobalamin is
recommended for those patients with abnormal renal function.

Table 1.   Indirect SNP Cerebral Effects

Cyanide	Hypoxia
Rebound Hypertension	Edema
↑ Cerebral Blood Flow	↑ ICP
↑ CSF CN	Hypoxia
Platelet Changes	Hematoma
Thiocyanate	↑ $CMRO_2$
↑ Pulmonary Shunting	Hypoxia

Thiocyanate increases when renal function is compromised, and produces abnormal central nervous system (CNS) activity.

Rebound hypertension occurs following abrupt discontinuance of SNP and results from increased plasma renin activity (PRA) from either ischemic or dilated renal vessels. Gradual SNP discontinuance, preoperative propranolol, and converting enzyme inhibitors will attenuate this response until increased PRA returns to normal (plasma half-life is 30 minutes).

Intracranial pressure (ICP) is increased in patients with low intracranial compliance as SNP dilates cerebral vessels and cerebral blood volume increases. Prior hyperventilation, steroids, and sedatives may improve compliance and allow SNP administration before opening the dura. Abnormal blood coagulation occurs after SNP induced platelet disintegration and inhibition of platelet aggregation. Hypothyroidism may result from thiocyanate interference with thyroid iodide trapping mechanisms.

Nitroglycerine (TNG) directly dilates capacitance vessels, has a short half-life, no toxic metabolites, and does not increase PRA. Resistance to TNG has been reported in certain patients receiving nonvolatile anesthetic techniques. Intracranial pressure increases in patients with low compliance contraindicating TNG use prior to dural opening unless prior hyperventilation, steroids, diuretics or sedatives have been administered (Table 2).

Trimethaphan is the only ganglionic blocker available in the United States. Sympathetic ganglia are blocked resulting in resistance and capacitance vessel relaxation and usually decreased arterial pressure. Its short plasma half-life makes for easy control. Histamine release has been reported to cause bronchospasm. Myoneural blockade has also been reported after trimethaphan because of its chemical resemblance to neuromuscular blocking drugs. Trimethaphan is recommended for MAP reductions above 50 torr as electroencephalogram (EEG) burst suppression, slowing and high voltage wave activity associated with increased brain lactate concentration occur at a MAP of 50 torr. These abnormalities have not been reported after SNP, TNG, or halothane induced MAPs of 50 torr (Table 3).

Hypotension is also produced by increasing inspired halothane, enflurane, or isoflurane concentration. Decreased blood pressure results primarily from myocardial depression and varying decreases in

Table 2. Indirect TNG Effects

↑ CBF	↑ ICP
↑ Pulmonary Shunting	↑ Hypoxia

Table 3. Direct Trimethaphan Cerebral Effects

↑ Lactate
↑ Postoperative Neurological Deficits
Abnormal EEG

---

total peripheral vascular resistance. Control is less easy than with
the previously discussed drugs. Potential adverse effects include
autoregulatory loss of vital organ blood flow, reduction in cerebral
perfusion pressure (CPP) as MAP decreases, and ICP increase in
patients with intracranial masses and increased cerebral edema. In
addition, anaerobic halothane metabolites may lead to hepatic cell
death.

Newer drugs, such as the calcium channel blockers and phentolamine, may have better characteristics as hypotensive drugs for use
in neurosurgical patients.

MECHANICAL MANEUVERS

Alterations in body position, mechanical ventilation, and heart
rate can be used in conjunction with the previously described drugs
to obtain the desired hypotensive level. These mechanical maneuvers
when properly used will decrease the total dose of potentially toxic
drugs necessary for maintenance of hypotension.

MONITORING

Routine monitoring should include the electrocardiogram (ECG)
with a V_5, blood pressure (BP) cuff, temperature probe, esophageal
stethoscope, and Foley, central venous (CVP), and arterial catheters.
In addition, a balloon-tipped flow directed thermodilution catheter
is helpful for pulmonary artery pressure (PAP) and pulmonary capillary wedge pressure (PCWP) measurement and cardiac output (CO) calculation.

Electrocardiographic monitoring is necessary during induced
hypotension to detect rhythm disturbances. Myocardial ischemia can
be detected with reasonable certainty by monitoring V_5. If ST segment changes occur, blood pressure should be adjusted accordingly if
arterial oxygenation and pH are normal.

A sphygmomanometer is helpful for determining the accuracy of
indwelling arterial catheter transduced values when placed on the
same arm or during periods of equipment malfunction.

Temperature monitoring is especially important when hypotension is induced, since body heat dissipates more rapidly from dilated vessels. Lowered body temperature may decrease the effectiveness of vasodilators and increase dose requirements if compensatory vasoconstriction occurs. Rectal or mid-esophageal temperature measurement reflects core temperature.

Decreases in urinary volume may indicate decreased renal perfusion and the need for higher blood pressure. Ionic and fluid replacement should be adequate prior to blood pressure level adjustment.

Central venous pressure monitoring prior to induced hypotension aids in assessing adequacy of effective circulating blood volume. Greater hypotensive response will be seen in hypovolemic patients at the onset of deliberate hypotension.

Direct indwelling arterial catheters are necessary for continuous blood pressure monitoring and determination of arterial blood gas values. Radial, femoral, or brachial arteries are suitable for short-term cannulation. The temporal and dorsalis pedis arteries can be used but cannulation may be difficult to achieve and maintain because of their small diameter. After proper testing for patency of the palmar arch, radial artery cannulation is preferable over other arteries.

Pulmonary artery pressure, PCWP, and calculation of CO are used to monitor fluid status, left heart function (especially in patients with ischemic or valvular heart disease), and to allow measurement of mixed venous oxygen tension ($P\bar{v}O_2$). Increase in $P\bar{v}O_2$ at low MAP may indicate decreased tissue perfusion and oxygen extraction from hemoglobin.

DIRECT CEREBRAL EFFECTS

Induced hypotension ideally should decrease CPP without significantly decreasing cerebral blood flow (CBF). This occurs when circulating blood volume and CO remain near normal as cerebrovascular resistance (CVR) decreses.

Cerebral blood flow will not support cerebral metabolism ($CMRO_2$) when mean CPP falls below 40 torr. Cerebral blood flow less than 18 ml/100 g/min occurs at 40 torr CPP. Higher levels of CPP and CBF are required to maintain $CMRO_2$ in patients with chronic hypertension or altered autoregulation. Lower CPP and CBF value may be permissible when anesthetic drugs suppress $CMRO_2$.

Lower limits of CPP and CBF necessary to maintain $CMRO_2$ have been determined in animals and humans by monitoring brain electrical activity (EEG), brain high energy substances and metabolites, and regional CBF (rCBF) measurements.

Brain electrical activity can be monitored with a multichannel EEG, which is a reliable method of diagnosing regional ischemia. Generally, EEG abnormalities occur when CBF falls below 18 ml/100 g/min or CPP falls below 40 torr. Trimethaphan-induced hypotension, however, produces EEG abnormalities at MAPs of 50 torr (Figure 1).

Brain energy substances - adenosine triphosphate, phospho-creatinine, glucose, glucose-6-phosphate and alpha-keto-glutarate - decrease when CBF is inadequate. Increasing concentration of brain lactate, pyruvate, and lactate/pyruvate ratio indicate brain ischemia and increased glycolysis. Decreases in brain energy substances and increases in glycolytic products occur when MAP reduction less than 50 torr is induced by SNP, trimethaphan, halothane, or hemorrhage in animals.

Regional CBF can be measured utilizing radioactive isotopes. These measurements are difficult to achieve in the operating room with the cranium open.

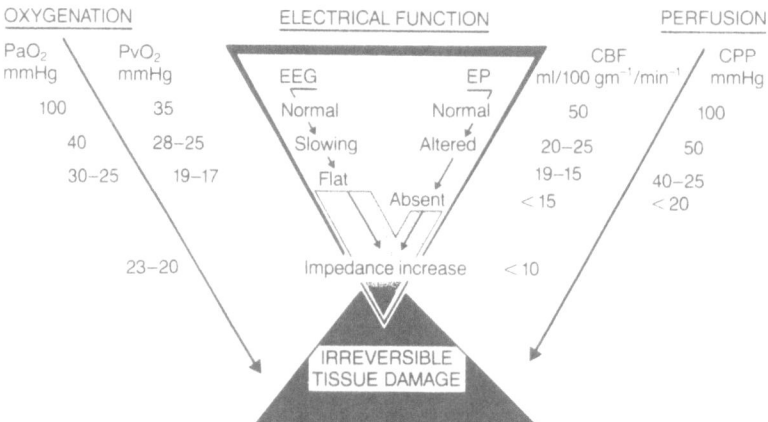

Fig. 1.   Threshold for changes in brain electrical activity. The shaded area at the bottom of the triangle represents a current deficiency in the neuroelectric monitoring capabilities. A gap exists between the last currently measurable electrical changes and the development of irreversible tissue damage. During arterial hypoxia brain oxygen extraction, CBF and CPP are presumed to increase as a normal physiologic response to oxygen deprivation. Oxygen extraction also increases when CBF and CPP are reduced. (from Shapiro H.M, 1978 ASA Refresher Course Lectures, Lecture No.109, p.12).

Maintenance of flow is critical when blood oxygen content is low. Decreases in arterial oxygen tension (PaO_2) below 40 torr with normal CBF results in increased metabolites suggestive of ischemia but little change in brain energy substances. As CBF decreases further, evidence of brain energy substance depletion and progressive ischemia occur.

During induced hypotension alterations in arterial carbon dioxide (CO_2) affects cerebral metabolism (MAP 50 torr). As $PaCO_2$ increases above 45 torr, brain energy substance concentration progressively decreases and lactate, pyruvate, and lactate/pyruvate ratios increase. Hypocarbia ($PaCO_2$ less than 25 torr) with hypotension (MAP of 50 torr) produces similar metabolic effects.

SUMMARY

Mean arterial pressure can be reduced to 50 torr safely in most patients. Brain energy substances and metabolic breakdown products are not altered by the hypotensive drugs previously discussed except for trimethaphan at these pressures. Higher MAPs are necessary in hypertensive patients with altered autoregulation and in brain regions compressed by masses. Cerebral blood flow must be maintained near normal during hypoxemia. Arterial carbon dioxide tension should be 35 to 45 torr during induced hypotension. Most of the cerebral effects of deliberate hypotension result from secondary atrogenic, physiologic, or pharmacologic effects of the drugs themselves.

REFERENCES

Abel, F. L., and Waldhausen, J., 1968, Influence of posture and passive tilting on venous return and cardiac output, Am.J.Physiol., 215:1058.

Boyan, C. P., 1953, Hypotensive anesthesia for radical pelvic and abdominal surgery, AMA Arch.Surg., 67:803-812.

Brunschwig, A., 1962, Hypotensive anesthesia, Am.J.Surg., 83:1-2.

Casthely, P., Lear, S., and Cottrell, J. E., Intrapulmonary shunting during induced hypotension, Anesth.Analg. (in press).

Chiarello, M., Gold, M. K., and Leinbach, R. C., 1976, Comparison between the effects of nitroprusside and nitroglycerin on ischemic injury during acute myocardial infarction, Circulation, 54:766-773.

Cottrell, J. E., Casthely, P. A., and Brodie, J. D., 1978, Prevention of nitroprusside-induced cyanide toxicity with hydroxocobalamin, N.Eng.J.Med., 298:809-811.

Cottrell, J. E., Gupta, B., and Turndorf, H., 1980, Induced hypotension, in: "Anesthesia and Neurosurgery," J. E. Cottrell and H. Turndorf, eds., C. V. Mosby, St. Louis, pp.387-400.

Cottrell, J. E., Illner, P., and Kittay, M. J., 1980, Rebound hyper-
    tension after sodium nitroprusside-induced hypotension,
    Clin.Pharm.Ther., 27:228-231.

Cottrell, J. E., Patel, K., and Casthely, P. A., 1981, Cerebrospinal
    fluid cyanide after nitroprusside infusion in man,
    Can.Anaesth.Soc.J., 28:228-231.

Cottrell, J. E., Patel, K., and Casthely, P. A., 1978, Nitroprusside
    tachyphylaxis without acidosis, Anesthesiology, 49:141-142.

Cottrell, J. E., Patel, K., and Ransohoff, J. R., 1978, Intracranial
    pressure changes induced by sodium nitroprusside in patients
    with intracranial mass lesions, J.Neurosurg., 48:328-331.

Cottrell, J. E., Gupta, B., and Rappaport, H., 1980, Intracranial
    pressure during nitroglycerin-induced hypotension,
    J.Neurosurg., 53:309-311.

Cottrell, J. E., and Turndorf, H., 1978, Intravenous nitroglycerin,
    Am.Heart.J., 96:550-553.

Davies, D. W., Kadar, D., and Steward, D. J., 1975, A sudden death
    associated with the use of sodium nitroprusside for induction
    of hypotension during anaesthesia, Can.Anaesth.Soc.J.,
    22:547-552.

Eckenhoff, J. E., Enderby, G. E. H., and Larson, A., 1963, Pulmonary
    gas exchange during deliberate hypotension, Br.J.Anaesth.,
    35:750-759.

Enderby, G. E. H., 1961, A report on mortality and morbidity follow-
    ing 9107 hypotensive anaesthetics, Br.J.Anaesth., 33:109-113.

Gardner, W. J., 1946, The control of bleeding during operation by
    induced hypotension, JAMA, 132:572-574.

Giffin, J. P., Thantun, E., Shwiry, B., and Cottrell, J. E., 1981,
    Effects of phentolamine on intracranial pressure, (Abstract),
    Anesthesiology, 55(3):A234.

Grundy, B. L., Nash, C. L., and Brown, R. H., 1979, Deliberate hypo-
    tension for scoliosis fusion, Anesthesiology, 51:S78.

Fahmy, N. R., 1978, Nitroglycerin as a hypotensive drug during
    general anesthesia, Anesthesiology, 49:17-20.

Harp, J. R., and Wollman, H., 1973, Cerebral metabolic effects of
    hyperventilation and deliberate hypotension, Br.J.Anaesth.,
    45:256-262.

Kerber, R. E., Martins, J. B., and Marcus, M. L., 1979, Effect of
    acute ischemia, nitroglycerin and nitroprusside on regional
    myocardial thickening, stress, and perfusion, Circulation,
    60:121.

Khambatta, J. H., Stone, J. G., and Khan, E., Hypertension during
    anesthesia on discontinuation of sodium nitroprusside-induced
    hypotension, Anesthesiology, 51:127-130.

Keigh, J. M., 1975, The history of controlled hypotension,
    Br.J.Anaesth., 47:745-749.

Levin, R. M., Zadigian, M. E., and Hall, S. C., 1980, The combined
    effect of hyperventilation and hypotension on cerebral oxygen-
    ation in anaesthetized dogs, Can.Anaesth.Soc.J., 27:264-273.

Little, D. M. Jr., 1955, Induced hypotension during anesthesia and
    surgery, Anesthesiology, 16:320-332.
Magness, A., Yashon, D., and Locke, G., 1973, Cerebral function
    during trimethaphan induced hypotension, Neurology, 23:506.
Mehta, P., Mehta, J. and Miale, T. D., Nitroprusside lowers platelet
    count, N.Eng.J.Med., 299:1134.
Michenfelder, J. D., and Theye, R. A., 1977, Canine systemic and
    cerebral effects of hypotension induced by hemorrhage, tri-
    methaphan, halothane, or nitroprusside, Anesthesiology,
    46:188-195.
Michenfelder, J. D., and Tinker, J. H., 1977, Cyanide toxicity and
    thiosulfate protection during chronic administration of sodium
    nitroprusside in the dog, Anesthesiology, 47:441-448.
Needleman, P., Jakschik, B., and Johnson, E. M., Jr., 1973,
    Sulfhydryl requirement for relaxation of vascular smooth
    muscle, J.Pharm.Exp.Ther., 198:324-331.
Nourok, D. S., Glassock, R. J., and Solomon, D. H., 1964, Hypothy-
    roidism following prolonged sodium nitroprusside therapy,
    Am.J.Med.Sci., 248:129-138.
Page, I. H., Corcoran, A. C., and Dustan, H. P., 1955, Cardiovascular
    actions of sodium nitroprusside in animals and hypertensive
    patients, Circulation, 11:188-198.
Pffeiderer, T., 1972, Sodium nitroprusside, a very potent platelet
    disaggregating substance, Acta Univ.Carol.(Med.Mongr)(Praha),
    53:247.
Posner, M. A., Tobey, R. E., and McElroy, H., 1976, Hydroxocobalamin
    therapy of cyanide intoxication in guinea pigs,
    Anesthesiology, 44:157-160.
Shanahan, R., 1973, The determination of sub-microgram quantities of
    cyanide in biological materials, J.Foren.Sci.Soc., 18:25-30.
Siesjo, B. K., Norberg, K., and Ljunggren, B., 1975, in: "A basis and
    practice of neuroanesthesia," E. Gordon, ed., Excerpta Medica,
    New York, pp.71.
Siesjo, B. K., and Zwetnow, N. N., 1970, The effect of hypovolemic
    hypotension on extra and intracellular acid-base parameters
    and energy metabolites in the rat brain, Acta Physiol.Scan.,
    79:114-124.
Smith, A. L., and Marque, J. J., 1976, Anesthetics and cerebral
    edema, Anesthesiology, 45:64-72.
Smith, R. D., and Kruszyna, H., 1974, Nitroprusside produces cyanide
    poisoning via a reaction with hemoglobin, J.Pharm.Exp.Ther.,
    191:557-563.
Stoyka, W. W., and Schutz, H., 1975, The cerebral response to sodium
    nitroprusside and trimethaphan controlled hypotension,
    Can.Anaesth.Soc.J., 22:275-283.
Tark, M., Anderson, M. A., and Teat, D., 1974, A simplified technique
    for measuring blood cyanide levels following nitroprusside
    infusion, Scientific Program Abstracts, Int.Anesth.Res.Soc.,
    p.68.

Thiagarajah, S., Tanaka, R., Marmarou, A., and Shulman, K., 1980,
    Evaluation of intracranial pressure dynamics in the cat during
    verapamil induced hypotension, Abstract, 1980 SNANSC Annual
    Meeting.
Thompson, G. E., Miller, R. D., and Stevens, W. C., 1978, Hypotensive
    anesthesia for total hip arthroplasty: a study of blood loss
    and organ function (brain, heart, liver and kidney),
    Anesthesiology, 48:91-96.
Tinker, J. H., and Michenfelder, J. D., 1976, Sodium nitroprusside:
    pharmacology, toxicology, and therapeutics, Anesthesiology,
    45:340-354.
Trembly, N. A. G., Davies, D. W., and Volgyesi, G., 1977, Sodium
    nitroprusside; factors which attenuate its action; studies
    with the isolated gracilis muscle of the dog, Can.Anaesth.
    Soc.J., 25:641-650.
Turner, J. M., Powell, D., and Gibson, R. M., 1977, Intracranial
    pressure changes in neurosurgical patients during hypotension
    induced with sodium nitroprusside or trimethaphan,
    Br.J.Anaesth., 49:419-425.
Van Dyke, R. A., 1978, Anesthetic biotransformation, ASA Annual
    Refresher Course Lectures, p.120.
Vesey, C. J., Cole, P. V., and Simpson, P. J., 1976, Cyanide and
    thiocyanate concentrations following sodium nitroprusside
    infusion in man, Br.J.Anaesth., 48:651-660.
Wang, H. H., Liu, L. M. P., and Katz, R. L., 1977, A comparison of
    the cardiovascular effects of sodium nitroprusside and
    trimethaphan, Anesthesiology, 46:40-48.

AUTOREGULATION OF CEREBRAL BLOOD FLOW:

EFFECTS OF HYPOTENSIVE DRUGS

W. Fitch, J. D. Pickard,
D. I. Graham and I. Arendt

University Departments of Anesthesia, Neurosurgery
and Neuropathology, University of Glasgow and the
Wellcome Surgical Institute, University of Glasgow
Glasgow, Scotland

The relationship between cerebral blood flow and the pressure perfusing the brain is of paramount importance in situations as diverse as hypovolemic shock, controlled or inadvertent hypotension during anesthesia and surgery, and in situations in which intracranial pressure is increased. The remarkable stability of the blood flow through the brain despite moderate variations in perfusion pressure was demonstrated in the early studies (Lassen, 1964; Harper, 1966), and the phenomenon of autoregulation was characterized. More recent investigations (Strandgaard et al., 1974; Fitch et al., 1976) delineated those values of mean arterial pressure beyond which the autoregulation of the cerebral circulation was ineffective and the basic pattern of the pressure flow relationship was established.

"Hypotensive" drugs are used widely in anesthesia and intensive care in the management of episodes of systemic hypertension and in the production of deliberate decreases in systemic arterial pressure. Their rational application depends largely on an appreciation of the pharmacological properties of the drugs themselves and on an awareness of how decreases in systemic arterial pressure affect the major organs. Their use during neurological surgery depends, in addition, on an understanding of those alterations to the basic physiological relationship between systemic arterial pressure and flow through the brain brought about by the presence of intracranial pathology.

The results to be presented below have been taken from a number of investigations in the anesthetized baboon in which systemic arterial hypotension was produced by the administration of increasing concentrations of several "hypotensive" agents - halothane, sodium nitroprusside and trinitroglycerine.

METHODOLOGY

The salient aspects of the methodology are presented here: the details have been described previously (Fitch et al., 1976; Boisvert et al., 1979; Pickard et al., 1980). The effects of progressive, graded hypotension on the pressure/flow relationship of the cerebral circulation were investigated in intact baboons (group A) and in similar animals one week after the induction of an artificial subarachnoid hemorrhage (group B). In this latter group, fresh autogenous blood (0.75 ml kg^{-1}) was injected into the suprachiasmatic cistern via a needle inserted percutaneously through the optic foramen.

Young adult baboons (8 - 15 kg), tranquillized with phencyclidine 12 mg i.m., were anesthetized with thiopentone 7.5 mg kg^{-1} i.v. and nitrous oxide 70 per cent in oxygen, supplemented with phencyclidine 4 mg i.m. every 30 minutes. Suxamethonium 50 mg i.m. was administered every 30 minutes also. The animals were ventilated artificially and the minute volume of ventilation and the inspired oxygen concentration were adjusted as required to maintain physiological tensions of carbon dioxide and oxygen in arterial blood. Cerebral blood flow (CBF) was measured by external scintillation counting over the right parietal area following the intracarotid injection of 133-Xenon in saline.

Following the measurement of baseline values, mean arterial pressure (MAP) was decreased progressively in steps of approximately 10 mm HG by the administration of increasing concentrations of the drugs under study. CBF was assessed at each decrement in MAP. In those animals (in both groups) receiving nitroprusside or nitroglycerine, acute increases in MAP were induced by the intravenous infusion of angiotensin (while maintaining the infusion of the hypotensive agent) once MAP had reached approximately 60 mm Hg. CBF was measured at these points also.

RESULTS

Baseline values of mean arterial pressure, cerebral blood flow and arterial carbon dioxide tension, obtained before there was any change in systemic arterial pressure, were similar in each of the studies included in this presentation.

Group A (Intact Animals)

As MAP was decreased moderately by the administration of the various drugs, CBF either remained stable (halothane) or increased significantly (nitroprusside and nitroglycerine). Following more marked decreases in MAP flow became pressure passive, the lower

limits of "autoregulation" being 40 mm Hg (halothane), 65 mm Hg
(nitroprusside) and 80 mm Hg (nitroglycerine). Where administered,
the infusions of angiotensin restored MAP to its baseline value but
this acute increase in arterial pressure was accompanied by significant increases in CBF.

Group B (SAH Animals)

In this group of animals decreases in CBF were associated with
the administration of halothane and nitroprusside - as MAP was decreased step-wise. In contrast, nitroglycerine induced a marked
increase in flow not dissimilar to that obtained using the same drug
in the intact animals. Once again, the administration of angiotensin
demonstrated that, during the infusion of either nitroprusside or
nitroglycerine, CBF responded passively to acute increases in MAP.

DISCUSSION

These investigations have demonstrated (a) that the reactivity
of the cerebral circulation is altered in the presence of an artificial subarachnoid hemorrhage and (b) that the pattern of the
pressure/flow relationship is affected, not only by intracranial
pathology but also by the particular drug used to effect the decreases in systemic pressure. For example, nitroglycerine produced
the most marked increases in flow and consequently, the greatest
changes in intracranial pressure.

The impairment of autoregulation in animals with subarachnoid
hemorrhage is not surprising (Harper et al., 1972; Hashi et al.,
1972). However, the demonstration that autoregulation was affected
in the animals without intracranial pathology during the administration of drugs with direct vasodilating properties is interesting and
of clinical relevance. Under these circumstances any variations in
the systemic circulation, be they increases or decreases in pressure,
will be reflected in the cerebral circulation. Moreover, from a
purely physiological point-of-view the findings suggest that one
cannot assess the integrity of autoregulation by using such drugs to
effect the alterations in arterial pressure: the overall effect on
the cerebral circulation being the result of competition between
direct cerebral vasodilatation, decreases in perfusion pressure and
possible impairment of autoregulation.

Acknowledgement

These studies were supported by the Medical Research Council.

REFERENCES

Boisvert, D. P. J., Pickard, J. D., Graham, D. I., and Fitch, W.,
      1979, Delayed effects of subarachnoid haemorrhape on cerebral
      metabolism and the cerebrovascular response to hypercapnia in
      the primate, J.Neurol.Neurosurg.Psychiat., 42:892.
Fitch, W., Ferguson, G. G., Sengupta, J., Garibi, J., and Harper,
      A. M., 1976, Autoregulation of cerebral blood flow during
      controlled hypotension in baboons, J.Neurol.Neurosurg.
      Psychiat., 39:1014.
Harper, A. M., 1966, Autoregulation of cerebral blood flow:
      influence of the arterial blood pressure on the blood flow
      through the cerebral cortex, J.Neurol.Neurosurg.Psychiat.,
      29:398.
Harper, A. M., Deshmukh, V. D., Sengupta, D., Rowan, J. O., and
      Jennett, W. B., 1972, The effect of experimental spasm on the
      CO_2 response of cerebral blood flow in primates,
      Neuroradiology, 3:134.
Hashi, K., Meyer, J. S., Shinmaru, S., Welch, K. M. A., and Teraura,
      T., 1972, Changes in cerebral vasomotor reactivity to CO_2 and
      autoregulation following experimental subarachnoid hemorrhage,
      J.Neurol.Sci., 17:15.
Lassen, N. A., 1964, Autoregulation of cerebral blood flow,
      Circ.Research, 15:(Suppl.) 201.
Pickard, J. D., Tamura, A., Graham, D. I., and Fitch, W., 1980,
      Response of the cerebral circulation to sodium nitroprusside-
      induced hypotension in normal baboons and one week after
      subarachnoid haemorrhage, in: "Pathophysiology and Pharmaco-
      therapy of Cerebrovascular Disorders," E. Betz, J. Grote,
      D. Heuser and R. Wullenweber, eds., Verlag Gerhard Witzstrock,
      Baden-Baden, Koln.
Strandgaard, S., MacKenzie, E. T., Sengupta, D., Rowan, J. O.,
      Lassen, N. A., and Harper, A. M., 1974, Upper limit of
      autoregulation of cerebral blood flow in the baboon,
      Circ.Research, 34:435.

THE DELETERIOUS EFFECT OF EXCESSIVE TISSUE

LACTIC ACIDOSIS IN BRAIN ISCHEMIA

S. Rehncrona

Laboratory of Experimental Brain Research
and Department of Neurosurgery
University Hospital of Lund, Lund, Sweden

The understanding of the basic series of events leading to brain cell damage and failure of postischemic neurological recovery is essential for the possibilities of taking adequate measures for brain protection in patients that run the risk of critical cerebral ischemia. Although extensively studied both clinically and experimentally (for literature see Siesjö, 1978; Rehncrona and Siesjö, 1981), the exact knowledge of those biochemical mechanisms that are directly responsible for the development of irreversible injury is relatively meagre. A mild to moderate decrease in tissue oxygen supply induces functional changes that are unrelated to any detectable deterioration of the cerebral energy state and most probably represent reversible changes in intercellular transmission. The more severe insults, leading to irreversible damage and cell death, have in common that energy production fails to keep pace with tissue energy demands, which results in a fast depletion of energy stores and energy failure. As a consequence of the lack of available energy (in the form of ATP) for the ionic pumps, ionic homeostasis is disrupted with loss of cellular K^+ and increase in intracellular Na^+, Cl^- and Ca^{2+} concentrations, often depicted as "membrane failure". Certainly these events are important for the development of cellular injury, but since they occur and are almost completed already within the first 2-4 minutes of complete ischemia, i.e. within a time period that is compatible with full neurological restitution, their exact relationship to irreversible damage is somewhat uncertain. Therefore other mechanisms operating either alone or in concert must also be considered.

Two facts from experimental research should be recalled. First, several investigations have shown that basic metabolic (like the energy state) and certain neurophysiological functions have a

potential capacity to recover even following prolonged (exceeding
15-30 min) ischemic periods at normothermia (Neely and Youmans, 1963;
Miller and Myers, 1970; Hossman and Kleihues, 1973; Ljunggren et al.,
1974b; Nordström et al., 1978a). Second, the degree of damage does
not always seem to be proportional to the degree of tissue hypoxia.
Thus, metabolic as well as neurophysiological recovery may be
significantly better following complete cerebral ischemia than
following similar periods of either severe hypoxia (Salford et al.,
1973a and b; Levy et al., 1975) or incomplete ischemia (Hossman and
Kleihues, 1973; Nordström et al., 1978b; Rehncrona et al., 1979b).
Obviously the remaining cerebral blood flow in the latter conditions
modifies the tissue response to oxygen deficiency in a detrimental
way.   Thus, we must consider the possibility that continued substrate
supply at a critically reduced oxygen availability leads to the
production of compounds, notably acid metabolites, which may affect
the capacity for postischemic recovery.

LACTATE ACCUMULATION IN DIFFERENT EXPERIMENTAL MODELS OF ISCHEMIA AND
HYPOXIA

     One of the first studies calling attention to the possibility of
a deleterious influence of accumulated lactic acid was published
about 20 years ago (Friede and van Houten, 1961).   These authors,
interested in postmortal morphological changes in brain tissue,
incubated cerebellar slices in a glucose medium.   They observed that
severe structural alterations developed concomittant to a continuous
drop in pH of the medium.   However, if glycolytic blockers were
added, pH remained unchanged and the cellular morphology well preserved.   The observation hints at the possibility that lactic acid,
formed by anaerobic glycolysis might be responsible for the more
severe structural changes observed in the first case.   Later, Myers
and collaborators (Myers and Yamaguchi, 1976, 1977; Myers, 1979)
found that administration of glucose to fasted animals (or using fed
experimental animals) markedly altered the final outcome and resulted
in increased brain damage in response to reversible circulatory
arrest.   Measurements of brain tissue lactate concentrations revealed
that levels exceeding 25-30 $\mu mol \cdot g^{-1}$ tissue during ischemia, related
to more severe damage.

     When the oxygen supply to the brain tissue is reduced below a
critical level, mitochondrial oxidative metabolism fails and extensive reduction of pyridine nucleotides occurs (Chance et al., 1962,
1964; for data on incomplete ischemia see also Rehncrona et al.,
1979a).   The redox change in the tissue will strongly favor pyruvate
reduction in the lactate dehydrogenase equilibrium leading to lactate
production and accumulation.   The level to which lactate accumulates
is dependent on the amount of glucose available for anaerobic glycolysis.   If the cerebral blood flow is totally interrupted (complete
ischemia) the rise in tissue lactate concentration is only determined

by the preishemic stores of glucose (and glycogen) in the tissue
(Ljunggren et al., 1974b). However, if ischemia is incomplete the
production of lactic acid also depends on the rate of the residual
blood flow, the duration of ischemia and, on the blood glucose concentration. Thus, in this situation, a continued delivery of substrates for glycosis may cause a much more severe tissue lactic
acidosis (lactate >25–30 $\mu mol \cdot g^{-1}$) as shown by Nordström and Siesjö
(1978).

Also in pronounced arterial hypoxia, a condition with preserved
tissue perfusion, glucose is continuously made available to the
hypoxic tissue. In the rat, severe tissue hypoxia can be induced by
combining a decreased arterial PO_2 (to about 20 mmHg) with unilateral
carotid artery occlusion. The latter procedure serving to restrict
the hypoxic hyperemia in the ipsilateral hemisphere. In experiments
with this model one observes a major deterioration of the tissue
energy state and increase in tissue lactate concentration to values
exceeding $25 \cdot \mu mol \ g^{-1}$ in more than 50% of the animals (Salford and
Siesjö, 1974). In the same model Salford et al. (1973a and b) found
deficient recovery of the tissue energy state as well as morphological signs of irreversible brain cell damage in the majority of
animals subjected to a 30 min reversible hypoxic period.

While the mdoel used for incomplete ischemia in the studies
quoted leaves a residual blood flow in brain cortical tissue below 5%
of normal (Nordström and Rehncrona, 1977), hypoxia with restricted
hyperemia is not encumbered with a decrease in CBF to values below
normal (Salford and Siesjö, 1974). However, both 30 min of pronounced incomplete ischemia and hypoxia with restricted hyperemia
obviously can be more harmful than a similar period of complete
cessation of the blood flow. Thus these results also favor the
hypothesis that continued substrate supply leading to excessive
tissue lactic acidosis has pathogenetic importance. Furthermore,
this hypothesis offers an explanation for the paradoxical finding
that a minimal residual blood flow actually can be harmful.

INFLUENCE OF DIFFERENT LACTATE CONCENTRATIONS IN THE ISCHEMIC BRAIN
UPON POSTISCHEMIC RECOVERY

In a recent series of experiments we have further tested the
hypothesis that the degree of ischemic tissue lactic acidosis is
critical for the possibility of postischemic recovery (Rehncrona
et al., 1980, 1981; Kalimo et al., 1981). The experiments were
performed in artificially ventilated rats under light nitrous oxide
anesthesia. Pronounced incomplete ischemia was induced by bilateral
carotid artery clamping combined with hypovolemic hypotension (mean
arterial blood pressure of 50 mmHg). After a 30 min ischemic period
recirculation was obtained by removal of the artery clamps and
normalization of the blood pressure. In order to vary lactic acid

production during ischemia all animals were deprived of food (but not
of water) during 16–24 hours before the experiment. In one group of
animals a glucose solution was infused i.v. 15 min before induction
of ischemia, while other experimental groups were given either a
similar volume of a physiological saline solution prior to ischemia
or a glucose solution only during the recirculation phase. Without
glucose pretreatment, the blood glucose concentration remained
slightly subnormal during ischemia (4–6 $\mu mol \cdot ml^{-1}$) but normalized in
the recirculation phase. Glucose pretreatment caused an increase in
blood glucose concentration to 25–35 $\mu mol \cdot ml^{-1}$ during ischemia and
these animals remained hyperglycemic during the subsequent recirculation phase. All animals had flat EEG during the ischemic period
and there were no responses to somatosensory stimulation. As evaluated from brain cortical concentrations of high energy phosphates,
ischemia caused a similar (and total) derangement of the cerebral
energy state in all experimental groups (cf. Figure 1). However, the
amount of accumulated lactate differed. Thus in saline–treated
animals tissue lactate concentration increased to around 15 $\mu mol \cdot g^{-1}$,
while glucose pretreatment caused the lactate concentration to rise
to around 35 $\mu mol \cdot g^{-1}$.

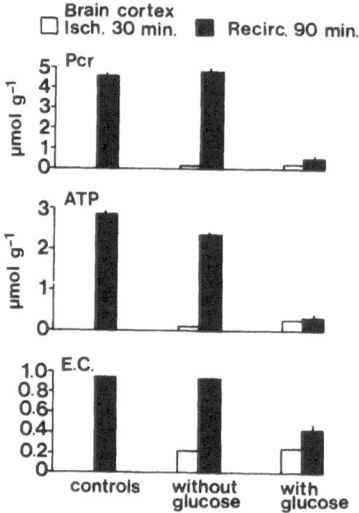

Fig. 1.   The recovery of cerebral energy state following pronounced
          incomplete ischemia, induced in fasted rats, with (ischemic
          lactate concentration about 15 $\mu mol \cdot g^{-1}$) and without
          (ischemic lactate conc. about 35 $\mu mol \cdot g^{-1}$) glucose pretreat-
          ment. PCr (Phosphocreatine), ATP (Adenosine triphosphate),
          EC = energy charge of the adenine nucleotide pool ([ATP] +
          0.5 [ADP])/([ATP] + [ADP] + [AMP]). Means ± SEM. (The
          Figure is based on values from Rehncrona et al., 1981).

As examplified in Figure 1 there was a remarkable difference in
postischemic metabolic recovery between the groups. Thus, the
animals infused with saline (low lactic acidotic group) recovered a
virtually normal cerebral energy state while hyperglycemic animals
did not show any metabolic recovery. Furthermore, the animals without glucose pretreatment recovered both spontaneous electrocortical
activity (normalized EEG pattern) as well as somatosensory evoked
responses (single shock and repetitive stimulation) while no recovery
of neuorphysiological parameters was observed in any of the animals
receiving glucose prior to ischemia (for details see Rehncrona et
al., 1981). Since hyperglycemia induced only during recirculation
failed to show any detrimental effect on recovery, the most plausible
explanation for the different outcome between the groups is the
difference in the level of accumulated lactate in the ischemic
tissue. Furthermore, as discussed by Dr. Kalimo in this volume (see
also Kalimo et al., 1981) morphological studies corroborate these
results by showing only mild and reversible cellular changes in the
saline-infused animals but widespread and irreversible cellular
damage in the animals rendered hyperglycemic before ischemia.

In correspondence to the results on incomplete ischemia,
metabolic recovery was shown to be impaired following 30 min of
complete ischemia if lactate production during ischemia was augmented
by increasing the preischemic stores of glucose substrates in the
tissue (Table 1). In these experiments the preischemic tissue substrate concentrations were increased by either hyperglycemia or by
combining hyperglycemia with hypercapnia, which increases the glucose
concentration ratio between intracellular water and blood.

Table 1. Differences in recovery of the cerebral energy
state following 30 min of complete brain ischemia
as related to tissue lactate concentrations
during the ischemic period. Values are means $\pm$
SEM of 4 animals. (Part of the material from
Rehncrona et al., 1981)

| | Ischemia 30 min | Recirculation 90 min | | |
	Lactate	ATP	E.C.	Lactate
Control	-------	2.80 +0.05	0.939 +0.002	2.64 +0.37
Normoglycemia Normocapnia	11.0 +0.6	2.08 +0.08	0.932 +0.002	3.85 +0.81
Hyperglycemia Normocapnia	22.3 +1.2	1.97 +0.05	0.913 +0.002	5.56 +0.87
Hyperglycemia + Hypercapnia	29.6 +2.0	1.40 +0.27	0.751 +0.09	14.2 +7.3

CONCLUDING REMARKS

From the data discussed here it seems reasonable to conclude
that the extent to which lactate accumulates in brain tissue during
ischemia is critical for the possibility of revival. Most probably
the deleterious effect of excessive production of lactate can be
explained by a concomittant severe fall in intracellular pH. Therefore, it is suggested that hyperglycemia should be avoided in clinical situations in which a reduced cerebral perfusion pressure may
provoke critical tissue ischemia and that efforts be made in search
for a clinically useful buffer solution efficient in the intracellular compartment of the brain.

REFERENCES

Chance, B., Cohen, P., Jöbsis, F., and Schoener, B., 1962,
     Intracellular oxidation - reduction states in vivo, Science,
     137:499-508.
Chance, B., Schoener, B., and Schindler, F., 1964, The intracellular
     oxidation - reduction state, in: "Oxygen in the Animal
     Organism," F. Dickens and E. Neil, eds., Pergamon Press,
     Oxford, pp.367-392.
Friede, R. L., and van Houten, W. H., 1961, Relations between
     post-mortem alterations and glycolytic metabolism in the
     brain, Exp.Neurol., 4:197-204.
Hossman, K. A., and Kleihues, P., 1973, Reversibility of ischemic
     brain damage, Arch.Neurol.(Chic.), 29:375-382.
Kalimo, H., Rehncrona, S., Söderfeldt, B., Olsson, Y., and Siesjö,
     B. K., 1981, Brain lactic acidosis and ischemic cell damage:2.
     Histopathology, J.Cereb.Blood Flow Metabol., 1:313-327.
Levy, D. E., Brierley, J. B., Silverman, D. G., and Plum, F., 1975,
     Brain hypoxia initially damages cerebral neurons,
     Arch.Neurol.(Chic.), 32:450-455.
Ljunggren, B., Norberg, K., and Siesjö, B. K., 1974a, Influence of
     tissue acidosis upon restitution of brain energy metabolism
     following total ischemia, Brain Res., 77:173-186.
Ljunggren, B., Ratcheson, R. A., and Siesjö, B. K., 1974b, Cerebral
     metabolic state following complete compression ischemia,
     Brain Res., 73:291-307.
Miller, J. R., and Myers, R. E., 1970, Neurological effects of
     systemic circulatory arrest in the monkey, Neurology
     (Minneap.), 20:715-724.
Myers, R. E., 1979, A unitary theory of causation of anoxic and
     hypoxic brain pathology, in: "Cerebral Hypoxia and its
     Consequences," S. Fahn, J. N. Davis, and L. P. Rowland, eds.,
     Adv.Neurol, Vol.26, Raven Press, New York, pp.195-213.
Myers, R. E., and Yamaguchi, S., 1977, Nervous system effects of
     cardiac arrest in monkeys. Preservation of vision,
     Arch.Neurol., 34:65-74.

Neely, W. A., and Youmans, J. R., 1963, Anoxia of canine brain
    without damage, JAMA, 183:1085-1087, (J.Amer.Med.Ass.)
Nordström, C. -H., and Rehncrona, S., 1977, Postischemic cerebral
    blood flow and oxygen utilization rate in rats anaesthetized
    with nitrous oxide or phenobarbital, Acta physiol.scand.,
    101:230-240.
Nordström, C. -H., Rehncrona, S., and Siesjö, B. K., 1978a,
    Restitution of cerebral energy state, as well as of glycolytic
    metabolites, citric acid cycle intermediates and associated
    amino acids offer 30 min of complete ischemia in rats anaesth-
    etized with nitrous oxide or phenobarbital, J.Neurochem.,
    30:479-486.
Nordström, C. -H., Rehncrona, S., and Siesjö, B. K., 1978b, Effects
    of phenobarbital in cerebral ischemia. Part two: Restitution
    of cerebral energy state, as well as of glycolytic metabol-
    ites, citric acid cycle intermediates and associated amino
    acids after pronounced incomplete ischemia, Stroke, 9:335-343.
Nordström, C. -H., and Siesjö, B. K., 1978, Effects of phenobarbital
    in cerebral ischemia. Part one: Cerebral energy metabolism
    during pronounced incomplete ischemia, Stroke, 9:327-335.
Rehncrona, S., Chance, B., and Austin, G., 1979a, Microheterogeneity
    of redox states in cerebral cortical tissue during hypoxia and
    ischemia, Adv.in Neurology, 26:325-333.
Rehncrona, S., Mela, L., and Siesjö, B. K., 1979b, Recovery of brain
    mitochondrial function in the rat after complete and incom-
    plete cerebral ischemia, Stroke, 10:437-446.
Rehncrona, S., Rosén, I., and Siesjö, B. K., 1980, Excessive cellular
    acidosis: an important mechanism of neuronal damage in the
    brain? Acta Physiol.Scand., 110:435-437.
Rehncrona, S., Rosén, I., and Siesjö, B. K., 1981, Brain lactic
    acidosis and cell damage. I. Biochemistry and neurophysiology,
    J.CBF.Metab., 1:297-311.
Rehncrona, S., and Siesjö, B. K., 1981, Metabolic and physiologic
    changes in acute brain failure, in: "Brain Failure and
    Resuscitation," A. Grenvik and P. Safar, eds., Churchill
    Livingstone, New York, pp.11-33.
Salford, L. G., Plum, F., and Brierley, J. B., 1973a, Graded
    hypoxiaoligemia in rat brain. II. Neuropathological alter-
    ations and their implications, Arch.Neurol., 29:234-238.
Salford, L. G., Plum, F., and Siesjö, B. K., 1973b, Graded
    hypoxiaoligemia in rat brain. I. Biochemical alterations and
    their implications, Arch.Neurol., 29:227-233.
Salford, L. G., and Siesjö, B. K., 1974, The influence of arterial
    hypoxia and unilateral carotid artery occlusion upon regional
    blood flow and metabolism in the rat brain,
    Acta Physiol.Scand., 92:130-141.
Siesjö, B. K., 1978, Brain Energy Metabolism, John Wiley & Sons,
    Chichester - New York - Brisbane - Toronto.

INTERACTION BETWEEN BLOOD GLUCOSE LEVEL, DEGREE OF CEREBRAL TISSUE
ACIDOSIS AND CELLULAR K$^+$ RELEASE UNDER CRITICAL CORTICAL FLOW
CONDITIONS

D. Heuser, H. Guggenberger, H. Heinle*, and F. Braig

Department of Anesthesia and
*Institute of Physiology (I)
University of Tübingen, FRG

INTRODUCTION

     Substantial evidence indicates that brain glucose concentration
at the moment of cerebral ischemic injury may be one of the most
important factors that affects severity of cell damage in central
nervous structures. Since glucose is the main substrate of cerebral
energy metabolism, it seems to be unquestionable that severe lactacidosis resulting from anaerobic glycolysis may be the culprit of
postischemic cell necrobiosis (Lindenberg, 1963; Myers, 1979;
Rehncrona et al., 1980; Kalimo et al., 1981; Rehncrona et al., 1981).
The correctness of this assumption has initially been shown in animal
studies demonstrating severe morphological cell damage following
cerebral ischemic injury in hyperglycemic animals) Myers and
Yamaguchi, 1977; Pulsinelli et al., 1980; Kalimo et al., 1981),
whereas cell damage in hypoglycemic animals was less pronounced and
of different morphological character (Agardh et al., 1981). With
regard to functional and metabolic recovery similar results have been
published (Siemkowiecz and Hansen, 1978, 1981; Rehncrona et al.,
1981) indicating worse outcome of total ischemia under conditions of
increased preischemic glucose availability in comparison to normoglycemia. Similar results in clinical studies have been obtained from
stroke-injured patients who demonstrated worse clinical outcome under
conditions of increased blood glucose levels prior to the ischemic
event (Pulsinelli et al., 1980).

     In the light of the above findings, there is no question that
the problem of imminent cerebral lactacidosis may be of considerable

The study was supported by a grant from the Deutsche Forschungs-
gemeinschaft He 1101/3-2.

significance in the course of the anesthetic management of patients with disturbed glucose metabolism prior to intraoperative conditions with potentially reduced cerebral blood flow, e.g. open heart surgery, intracranial interventions, severe head injuries as well as during controlled hypotension.

The aim of the present animal study was to directly and continuously analyze the extent and possible enhancement of cerebral extracellular acidosis due to increased preischemic glucose availability in a model of severe incomplete regional ischemia. Furthermore, the membrane-stabilizing effect of high glucose levels, which can be measured in terms of extracellular K^+ activities (Artru and Michenfelder, 1981; Astrup et al., 1981) and may be mediated by residual ATP generation during anaerobic glycolysis, was also investigated to see whether this effect may be pronounced enough to possibly counterbalance the detrimental effect of severe lactacidosis in cerebral tissue under the present experimental conditions.

EXPERIMENTAL PROTOCOL

Experiments were performed on 12 cats subjected to halothane (0.5 - 1.5% vol) anesthesia under relaxation and mechanical ventilation (N_2O/O_2 = 2:1). Mean arterial blood pressure as well as endexpiratory CO_2 content were recorded continuously. Blood gases and body temperature were checked intermittently and maintained at normal levels throughout the experiments. Extracellular H^+ and K^+ activities were measured continuously using ion-selective microelectrodes which were implanted - via a cranial window under stereomicroscopical observation - in an area of the cerebral cortex supplied from the middle cerebral artery (MCA). The pH electrodes were glass microelectrodes with tip diameters varying between 2 and 10 μm. They were constructed using a modification of the technique developed in our laboratory (Heuser, 1976). Calibration was performed in appropriate buffer solutions corrected for the NaCl-induced changes in junction potentials at the tip of the reference cell (Maas, 1971). Response time, slope, and stability varied within the range of commercially available pH electrodes (<1 sec; 53-59 mV/pH; <1 mV/h). The K^+ microelectrodes were designed using a modification of Walker's technique (1971): a commercially available liquid ion exchanger (Corning Code 477317) was sucked into the very tip of a siliconized pyrex glass pipette of 1-2 μm tip diameter and covered with 0.5 M KCl. As with the pH electrodes, we used chloridized silver wires as an internal reference. Calibration was performed in solutions of a mixture of KCl and NaCl and included constant cation molality of 150 mmoles/liter. An ordinary glass pipette drawn to a tip diameter of 1-2 μm and filled with 0.9% NaCl in 1% agar served as an external reference. Electrode potentials were recorded differentially against this "microreference" using operational amplifiers of high input impedance ($10^{12}\Omega$), whereas a second reference cell buried deeply in the neck muscles was used as a common ground for the system.

Critically reduced regional cerebral blood flow was induced by temporarily clipping the MCA or one of its cortical branches via a lateral approach. Clipping of ten minutes duration was performed three times in each animal. Prior to the second and third clipping, glucose was administered intravenously to obtain levels of 160 and 280 mg/100 ml (Table 1). Second and third clippings were not performed, however, until normal ionic equilibrium was reobtained, which usually required 20 to 30 minutes. Statistical evaluation of the results was performed using tests for non-gaussian distributed groups (e.g., Wilcoxon-Pratt).

RESULTS

I. Clipping of the middle cerebral artery causes a highly reproducible sequence of events in cerebral ion homeostasis characterized by progressively developing acidosis and an increase in extracellular K^+ activity (Figure 1). In contrast to the progressively increasing acidosis, cellular K^+ release usually occurs in three steps: 1) an initially slow progressive increase up to values of 8-10 mM; followed by, 2) a sudden K^+ release up to K^+ levels of 50-60 mM; 3) a third phase which is slow again and approaches peak levels of 70-80 mM.

Table 1. Local changes in cerebral extracellular cationic activities (H^+ and K^+) during severe incomplete regional ischemia (MCA clipping) under various degrees of preischemic glucose availability. The Wilcoxon-Pratt test was used for statistical evaluation

		initial values	normo-glycemia	moderate hyperglycemia	severe hyperglycemia
pH	Median	7.36	6.62	6.30	6.24
	Min.	7.14	5.90	5.87	5.70
	Max.	7.52	6.91	6.52	6.48
	n=11	└─── *** ───┘		└─── ** ───┘	
			└────────── * ──────────┘		
K^+	Median	3.8	41	45	39
[mM]	Min.	3.0	12	10	10
	Max.	5.0	80	75	70
	n=8	└── ** ──┘ └── * ──┘		└── * ──┘	
			└────────── * ──────────┘		
Glucose [mg/100 ml]	Mean ± SD	90.0 ± 13.6	90.6 ± 14.7	163.4 ± 21.6	277.8 ± 47.4

*p < 0.05   **p < 0.01   ***p < 0.001

However, it must be emphasized that K^+ leakage occurs only at cerebral blood flow levels below 10-14 ml/100 g·min., when electrical activity, measured as spontaneous EEG, is no longer detectable. The high reproducibility of these ionic shifts is demonstrated in Figure 1, which shows the effects of three clampings in a single animal.

II.   4) Reperfusion leads to normalization of the disturbed ionic equilibrium. K^+ levels usually normalize a bit more quickly than pH, and the time course of reattainment of normal ionic homeo-stasis can be modified by metabolic-depressive drugs (e.g., Etomidate).

III.   Administration of glucose significantly modifies the degree of ionic disequilibrium: a distinct enhancement of tissue acidosis occurs under moderate hyperglycemia (Figure 2), and an even more severe increase at very high glucose levels. This enhancement of tissue lactacidosis after glucose administration was observed in all but two of the animals. In these two exceptions, clipping ob-viously was not performed properly. Extracellular acidosis in the present model of incomplete cerebral ischemia was less than the level at normoglycemia in one animal which turned out to be hypoglycemic.

IV.   Potassium leakage from cells of the central nervous system is slightly modified by increased arterial glucose levels and seems to reflect a membrane-stabilizing effect (Figure 3). This could be

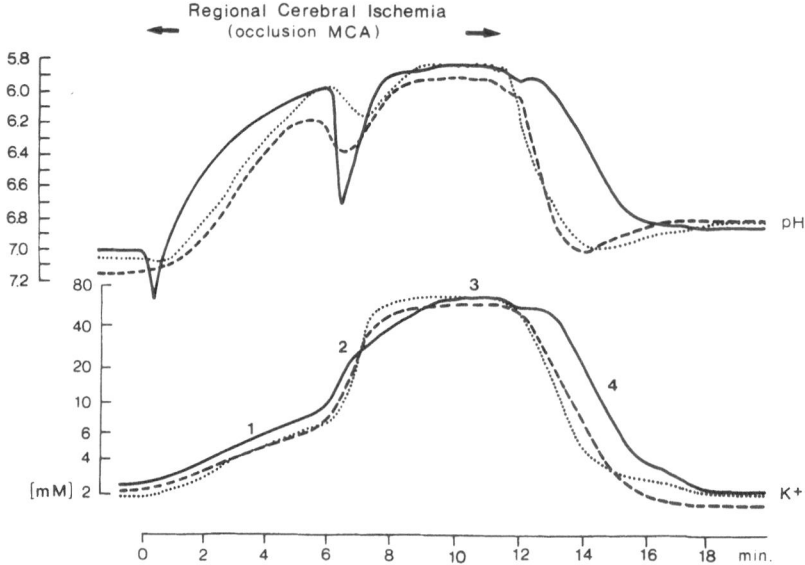

Fig. 1.   Changes in local extracellular H^+ and K^+ activities in the cerebral cortex of cats during critically reduced regional CBF (MCA clipping). The figure demonstrates the high re-producibility of the ionic changes in synoptic plots of three subsequent clampings in one animal. 1,2,3,4 see text.

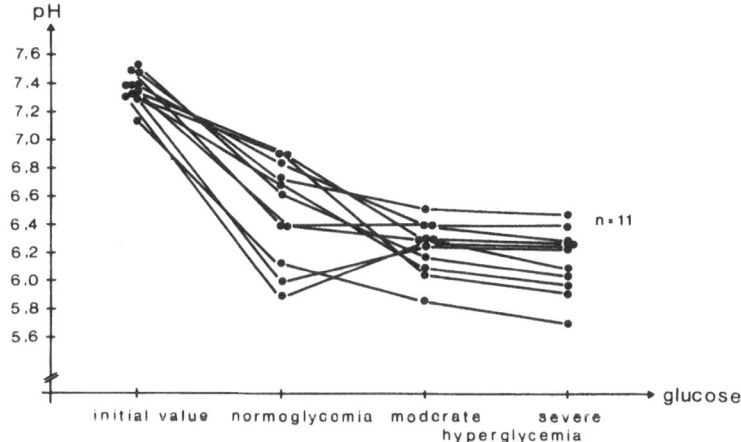

Fig. 2. Enhancement of local tissue acidosis in the cerebral cortex
of cats (n=11) due to increased preischemic glucose availability during severe incomplete regional ischemia (MCA
clipping), measured in terms of pH values.

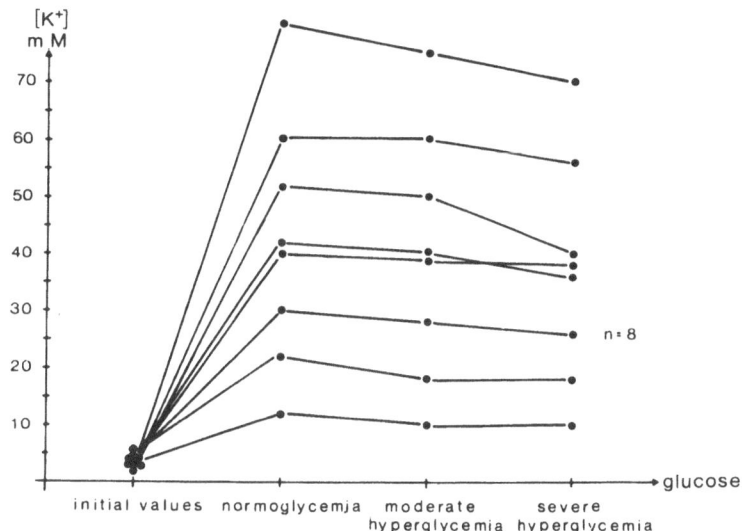

Fig. 3. Slight membrane-stabilizing effect of increased preischemic
glucose availability in cats (n=8), measured in terms of
peak values of extracellular K^+ activity during severe
incomplete ischemia (MCA clipping). The large scatter of K^+
changes reflects different degrees of focal ischemia at the
measuring sites.

due to residual ATP generation by continuous anaerobic glycolysis
maintained by the relatively increased glucose availability.

The statistic evaluation of the present results based on the
Wilcoxon-Pratt test is shown in Table 1.

DISCUSSION

The present experimental data confirm the notion that enhanced
severity of cerebral tissue acidosis due to increased cerebral availability of glucose at the moment of severe incomplete ischemia may
indeed contribute to more pronounced manifestation of neurological
deficits. Thus, the present results emphasize the necessity of
establishing approximately normal blood glucose levels prior to the
anesthetic management of those surgical patients subject to a risk of
major intraoperative reductions in cerebral perfusion, e.g. during
extracorporal circulation, intracranial interventions, and controlled
hypotension.

One question, however, has not yet been sufficiently answered:
since lactacidosis and cellular K^+ release always occurred simultaneously in the present experiments, one cannot discriminate as to
which metabolic event may be more detrimental to CNS cells membrane
failure or severe lactacidosis. It is unquestionable that the combination of both is most harmful; experiments designed to clearly
separate both effects would be helpful and are now in progress in our
laboratory. In light of the present experimental data, it seems
unlikely that the small membrane-stabilizing effect of high preischemic glucose availability under the present conditions of severe
incomplete ischemia could actually outweigh the disadvantages of
severe lactacidosis - a notion which has been confirmed in recent
morphological studies (Kalimo et al., 1981). Under conditions of
complete interruption of cerebral circulation, however, the membrane-
stabilizing effect seems to be more pronounced (Siemkowicz and
Hansen, 1981). Nevertheless, it should be emphasized that membrane
stabilization, as measured by maintained homeostatis in K^+ distribution, can also be achieved by other means, as has been suggested
recently (Artru and Michenfelder, 1981; Astrup et al., 1981). An
appropriate buffer solution suitable to maintaining normal intracellular H^+ activities has not yet been developed. Solving this
problem appears to be one of the urgent tasks facing future research
in the field.

REFERENCES

Agardh, C. D., Kalimo, H., Olsson, Y., and Siesjö, B. K., 1981,
        Hypoglycemic brain injury: metabolic and structural findings
        in rat cerebellar cortex during profound insulin-induced

hypoglycemia and in the recovery period following glucose administration, J.Cereb.Blood Flow Metabol., 1:71.

Artru, A. A., and Michenfelder, J. D., 1981, Anoxic cerebral potassium accumulation reduced by phenytoin: mechanisms of cerebral protection, Anaesth.Analg., 60:41.

Astrup, J., Sorsted, P., Gjerris, F., and Rahbeck Sørensen, H., 1981, Increase in extracellular potassium in the brain during circulatory arrest: effects of hypothermia, lidocaine and thiopental, Anaesthesiology, 55:256.

Heuser, D., 1976, Die potentiometrische Bestimmung von perivaskulären H^+ und K^+-Aktivitäten bei Untersuchungen der lokalen Regulation des cerebralen Gefäßwiderstandes. Habilitationsschrift, Tübingen.

Kalimo, H., Rehncrona, S., Söderfeldt, B., Olsson, Y., and Siesjö, B. K., 1981, Brain lactic acidosis and ischemic cell damage: 2. Histopathology, J.Cereb.Blood Flow Metabol., 1:313.

Lindenberg, R., 1963, Patterns of CNS vulnerability in acute hypoxaemia, including anaesthesia accidents, in: "Selective vulnerability of the brain in hypoxaemia," J. Schade and W. Menemy, eds., F. A. Davis Co., Philadelphia, :189.

Maas, A. H. J., 1971, pH determination in body fluids using a cell with an isotonic sodium chloride bridge, J.appl.Physiol., 30:248.

Myers, R. E., 1979, A unitary theory of causation of anoxic and hypoxic brain pathology, in: "Advances in Neurology 26. Cerebrial hypoxia and its consequences," S. Fahn, J. N. Davis, and L. P. Rowland, eds., Raven Press, New York, :195.

Myers, R. E., and Yamaguchi, S., 1977, Nervous system effects of cardiac arrest in monkeys, Arch.Neurol., 34:65.

Pulsinelli, W., Waldman, S., Sigsbee, B., Rawlinson, D., and Plum, F., 1980, Experimental hyperglycemia and diabetes mellitus worsen stroke outcome, in: "Pathophysiology and Pharmacotherapy of cerebrovascular disorders," E. Betz, J. Grote, D. Heuser, and R. Wüllenweber, eds., Verlag G. Witzstrock, Baden-Baden - Köln - New York :196.

Rehncrona, S., Rosen, J., and Siesjö, B. K., 1980, Excessive cellular acidosis: An important mechanism of neuronal damage in the brain? Acta Physiol.Scand., 110:435.

Rehncrona, S., Rosen, J., and Siesjö, B. K., 1981, Brain lactic acidosis and ischemic cell damage: 1. Biochemistry and Neurophysiology, J.Cereb.Blood Flow Metabol., 1:297.

Siemkowicz, E., and Hansen, A. J., 1978, Clinical restitution following cerebral ischemia in hypo-, normo- and hyper-glycemic rats, Acta neurol.Scand., 58:1.

Siemkowicz, E., and Hansen, A. J., 1981, Brain extracellular ion composition and EEG activity following 10 minutes ischemia in normo- and hyperglycemic rats, Stroke, 12:236.

Walker, J. L., 1971, Ion specific liquid ion exchanger microelectrodes, Anal.Chem., 43:89A.

Welsh, F. A., Ginsberg, M. D., Rieder, W., and Budd, W. W., 1980,
     Deleterious effect of glucose pretreatment on recovery from
     diffuse cerebral ischemia in the cat. II. Regional metabolic
     levels, Stroke, 11:355.

CONTROLLED HYPOTENSION IN NEUROANESTHESIA

P. J. Morris, D. Heuser* and D. G. McDowall

Department of Anesthesia
The University of Leeds, England
*Department of Anesthesia
University of Tübingen, FRG

Hypotensive techniques are frequently employed for major neuro-surgical operations. The rationale for the use of such techniques is based upon the observation that, in cases of intracerebral arterial aneurysm, the tension in the wall of the aneurysm can be reduced by lowering the systemic arterial pressure. Similarly, the blood flow to vascular tumors of the brain is supplied by blood vessels which have lost their capacity to autoregulate and the flow in such vessels can also be reduced by inducing systemic hypotension. The advantages to the surgeon of a locally-reduced blood flow in these instances will be obvious, allowing the clipping of a tense aneurysm and reducing hemorrhage during the dissection of a vascular tumor. However, hypotensive techniques carry the possibility of more widespread derangements in cerebral perfusion and the severity of these derangements may not only be related to the depth of hypotension, but may also be influenced by the drugs used to produce the hypotension.

Currently, the methods used to electively induce systemic arterial hypotension in neurosurgical anesthesia are based on the intravenous infusion of drugs having either a direct vasodilator action or a ganglion-blocking action, and the two most commonly used agents are sodium nitroprusside (NTP) and trimetaphan (TMP). NTP, a direct-acting vasodilator, and TMP, a ganglion-blocking agent, as might be expected from their different modes of action, have been shown to differ significantly in their influence on the cerebral circulation (Michenfelder and Theye, 1977; Maekawa et al., 1979). NTP maintains a higher cerebral blood flow (CBF) than TMP during hypotension, and this higher CBF is associated with a higher cortical surface oxygen tension.

In view of these known differences, it seemed possible that further disturbances might be produced in the cortex during hypotension, and we therefore examined the changes in cerebral extracellular fluid (ecf) ion homeostases which accompany the circulatory changes produced by NTP and TMP in an animal model using ion-selective microelectrodes.

Cats were anesthetized with a nitrous oxide, oxygen/halothane mixture and, after initial muscle relaxation with intramuscular (i.m.) suxamethonium 75 mg, the animals were intubated and ventilated to normocapnia. Neuromuscular blockade was maintained with i.m. pancuronium. The animals' body temperature was maintained between 37 and 39°C using warming blankets. The femoral artery and vein were cannulated bilaterally and catheters were passed into the abdominal aorta and inferior vena cava to allow mean arterial blood pressure (MABP) measurement, intermittent arterial blood sampling for blood gas analysis, intravenous (i.v.) fluid therapy and drug infusion. Each animal received i.v. Ringer's lactate solution 4 ml/kg^{-1}/hr^{-1}.

In order to measure regional cerebral blood flow (rCBF) the right lingual artery was exposed and catheterized through an incision beneath the mandible. The tip of the catheter was adjusted to lie at the junction of the lingual artery and the carotid artery. rCBF was subsequently measured by recording the wash-out of the β radiation from Krypton 85 (^{85}Kr) from the cortex following a 2 min infusion of ^{85}Kr in saline injected via the lingual artery cannula into the carotid artery. With the animal in the sphinx position, the muscles overlying the skull were excised through a mid-line scalp incision and bilateral parietal burr holes approximately 1.0-1.5 cm in diameter were made on the inter-auricular line 1 cm from the midline. The dura overlying the right cortex was opened and widely reflected to expose the underlying cortex, which was covered with a transparent plastic sheet impermeable to carbon dioxide (MELINEX® ICI). The clearance of ^{85}Kr from the cortex was measured using a Geiger-Müller tube placed over this burr hole. The dura overlying the left parietal cortex was also opened, but only wide enough to allow the implantation of three microelectrodes into the cortex.

Cortical ecf ion activities were measured in the cortex using ion-sensitive microelectrodes. The K$^+$ ion-selective electrode was manufactured from borosilicate glass capillaries 2 mm in diameter, drawn in an electrode puller to a tip diameter of 1-2 μm. The tubes were then exposed to the vapor of dimethylsiloxone and the tips were filled with Corning K$^+$ selective ion exchange resin. The tube was then filled from the open end with 0.5 molar K Cl and a silver/silver chloride (Ag/AgCl) wire was inserted into the electrode and sealed in place with dental wax, the end of the tube being left open.

Cortical ecf pH was measured with a glass microelectrode of tip diameter less than 10 μm, constructed using a modification of the

technique of Gebert (1972). Corning pH glass capillaries were drawn
to a tip diameter of less than 10 μm and such a capillary was then
fitted closely inside an insulating capillary consisting of a lead
glass tube of 2-3 mm external diameter drawn to the appropriate tip
shape. Under stereomicroscope vision, the lead glass capillary had
been broken off to allow the pH glass tip to protrude approximately
60 μm. Gentle heating in a microforge melted the lead glass capillary at the base of the pH glass tip to seal the latter in position.
Further heating of the pH glass tip was undertaken in order to melt
and seal the tip of the pH glass. When cool, the pH glass capillary
was broken off above the seal with the lead glass and the electrode
was filled with tris buffered 0.1 N hydrochloride acid at pH 7.20 and
an Ag/AgCl wire was sealed into the electrode using dental wax.

Reference electrodes consisted of a borosilicate glass tube of
2 mm diameter drawn to a tip diameter of 2 μm and filled with a gel
consisting of 0.9% sodium chloride solution containing 2% Agar. A
similar reference electrode of 2 mm diameter was implanted in the
neck. The ion-selective electrodes and micro reference electrode
were suspended from compliant springs made of fine copper wire and,
held in micromanipulators, they were implanted in the cortical mantle
to a depth of approximately 500 μm. The outputs of the ion-selective
electrodes were amplifed differentially against the two reference
electrodes so that changes in D.C. potential on the brain did not
influence observed values of K^+ and pH. D.C. differential amplifiers
with a high-input empedance (c.10^{14} Ω) were employed. Calibration of
the pH electrodes was carried out using appropriate buffers and the
K^+ selective electrodes were calibrated in solutions of K^+ in Na Cl
with K^+ concentrations of 1, 3, 5, 8, 10, 20 and 40 mM with the Cl^-
concentration being maintained at 150 mM, the cationic balance being
maintained at 150 mM, by Na^+. All electrodes were calibrated before
and after each experiment and results obtained were discarded if the
post-experiment calibration was inappropriate. For this reason K^+
measurements were obtained in 12 experiments and pH in 8 experiments.

Following electrode implantation 30 min was allowed for the
preparation to stabilize prior to control measurements being made.
Three control measurements of rCBF were made and the values for MABP,
ecf K^+, pH and $PaCO_2$ were recorded during each ^{85}Kr clearance. All
the animals then received i.v. practolol 0.2 mg/kg^{-1} and each animal
was randomly allocated to receive either an NTP or a TMP infusion.

In view of its toxicity, NTP was infused to a maximum dose of
1 mg/kg^{-1} and the dose limit for TMP was set at 10 mg/kg^{-1}. The BP
was lowered at a rate of 5 mm Hg·min^{-1} until a mean arterial blood
pressure (MABP) of 30-32 mm Hg was achieved, when a further dose of
practolol 0.1 mg/kg was given. This MABP was maintained for 30 min
and the MABP was lowered further to 26-28 mm Hg and held at this
level for a further 15 min. In order to achieve these levels of

hypotension without resorting to massive drug dosage, controlled arteriotomy was used. Blood withdrawal into a heparanized syringe from a femoral artery catheter was instituted when drug infusion at its maximum rate ceased to produce an appropriate fall in BP. Similar mean values of blood withdrawal were recorded in both the NTP and the TMP animals.

Comparison of means of recorded data was carried out using either the Student t test or the Wilcoxon-Rank Sum test, as appropriate.

Hypotension with both TMP and NTP was accompanied by a cortical ecf acidosis. With TMP the cortical ecf pH fell from a control value of 7.21 ± 0.05 to 5.85 ± 0.15. The fall in cortical ecf pH with NTP hypotension was from 7.16 ± 0.02 to 6.55 ± 0.18.

Table 1 shows the changes in mean values from control of MABP, rCBF, $PaCO_2$ and brain ecf K+. As expected from the previous work of Michenfelder and Theye (1977), hypotension with TMP produced a significant fall in rCBF and associated with this value of rCBF was a significant increase in cortical ecf K+.

Hypotension with TMP to the levels described produces cortical ischemia sufficient to impair the ability of the neuronal cell membrane to maintain its integrity with regard to K^+ ions. Metabolic energy is required for the Na^+/K^+ pump within the cell membrane, and failure of perfusion with TMP will result in failure of oxygen delivery and of carbon dioxide clearance. Although the latter effect might contribute to the worse cortical ecf acidosis recorded with TMP, the former would certainly encourage anaerobic metabolism with the production of an increasing tissue lactate concentration. The value for rCBF associated with K^+ release into the cortical ecf

Table 1. Mean Values ± S.E. for MABP, rCBF, $PaCO_2$ and K+

		MABP [mm Hg]	rCBF [ml $100g^{-1}min^{-1}$]	$PaCO_2$ [kPa]	Brain ecf K+ [mmol]
Control values	NTP	116 ± 8	67 ± 5	4.4 ± 0.2	3.3 ± 0.3
	TMP	104 ± 5	66 ± 6	4.4 ± 0.2	3.3 ± 0.3
Hypotensive values	NTP	27 ± 0.3	53*± 10	4.1 ± 0.2	4.6*± 0.7
	TMP	28 ± 1.0	16*± 5	5.0 ± 0.2	26.4*± 5.8

*Denotes a significant difference between NTP and TMP mean values ($p < 0.05$).

(Figure 1) is somewhat higher than the threshold values observed by
Astrup et al. in baboons (1977), and further work in cats by Heuser
and Astrup (Heuser – personal communication) demonstrated an rCBF
threshold for K^+ release similar to that in the baboons, thus making
a species difference unlikely. Methodological differences could
explain the discrepancy in observed rCBF threshold values, as both
Astrup et al. (1977) and Heuser and Astrup (Heuser – personal communication) employed a hydrogen (H_2) clearance technique using plat-
inum microelectrodes to record the H_2 wash-out. These microelectrodes were implanted in the boundary zones, i.e., implanted in an
area of cortex lying between the zones supplied by the anterior,
middle and posterior cerebral arteries. Although the ^{85}Kr clearance
was also recorded from the boundary zone, the counter averaged counts
from an area of cortex approximately 1 cm in diameter, and thus areas
of cortex potentially better-perfused were included in the counting
field, thus giving a higher average rCBF. Due to the high diffus-
ibility of H_2 it is also possible that the H_2 electrodes used in
other studies were influenced by white matter flow.

The cortical ecf acidosis observed during the NTP hypotension is
more difficult to explain, as the rCBF value measured at this time

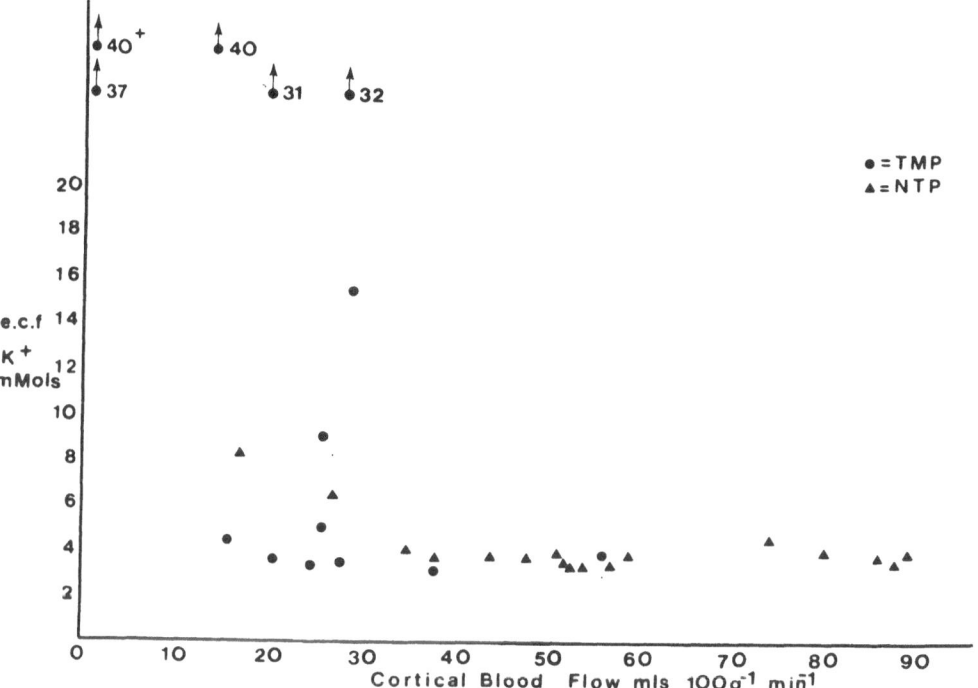

Fig. 1.   Threshold of rCBF for K^+ release into the cortical ecf
          during controlled hypotension induced with either
          Trimetaphan (TMP) or Sodium Nitroprusside (NTP).

was not ischemic, and was only moderately reduced from the control value. The minimal tissue carbon dioxide retention which would accompany such a small reduction in perfusion would not cause the observed fall in cortical ecf pH. A direct toxic effect of the NTP due to tissue cyanide giving rise to poisoning of the oxidative enzymes cannot be excluded as a possible cause for this acidosis, but seems unlikely as the total dose of NTP of 1 mg/kg^{-1} is just within the currently accepted limit. Oligemic hypotension has been shown to have a deleterious effect on both CBF and cerebral metabolism and the blood withdrawal in both groups of animals may have contributed to the abnormal acidosis.

NTP maintains rCBF during profound hypotension, with only moderate derangements in the ionic homeostasis of the cerebral ecf, whilst hypotension to similar values with TMP is associated with cerebral ischemia with more severe disturbance in the cerebral ecf ionic environment. If the human cerebral circulation behaves in similar fashion, it would appear that the direct vasodilator action of NTP holds advantages over TMP when profound hypotension is required during neurosurgery.

REFERENCES

Astrup, J., Symon, L., Branston, N. M., and Lassen, N. A., 1977, Cortical evoked potential and extracellular K+ and H+ at critical levels of brain ischemia, Stroke, 8:51-57.

Gebert, G., 1972, Die Messung von Na+, K+ und H+ - Aktivitäten im Gewebe mit Glasmikroelektroden, Arztl.Forsch., 26:379-385.

Maekawa, T., McDowell, D. G., and Okuda, Y., 1979, Brain-surface oxygen tension and cerebral cortical blood flow during hemorrhagic and drug-induced hypotension in the cat, Anesthesiology, 51:29-36.

Michenfelder, J. D., and Theye, R. A., 1977, Canine systemic and cerebral effects of hypotension induced by hemorrhage, trimetaphan, halothane or nitroprusside, Anesthesiology, 46:188-195.

MEMBRANE STABILIZATION IN THE ISCHEMIC BRAIN:

A MODE OF PROTECTION?

J. Astrup

Department of Neurosurgery
Copenhagen County Hospital at Hvidovre
2650 Hvidovre, Denmark

If cerebral circulatory arrest occurs, oxidative metabolism and hence almost all ATP production will cease. The cells rapidly become depleted of ATP, the energy-requiring processes such as ion transport are halted, the cells leak K^+ and take up Na^+, Cl^-, Ca^{2+} and water, and the membranes depolarize. This is the general scheme of events followed by all ischemic tissues, but the remarkable feature of the brain is the rapidity by which this occurs. Due to extreme leakiness of the cellular compartment in the brain the state of terminal ischemic membrane failure is reached in a matter of minutes, while it may take hours or even days for the passive ion leak fluxes to reach completion in other organs with tight membranes such as muscle, peripheral nerve, or erythrocytes.

The high rate of Na^+ and K^+ leak fluxes in ischemic brain suggests membrane leakiness and a high rate of leak fluxes of these ions also in normal non-ischemic brain in which the leak must be continuously counteracted by ATP-consuming NA^+-K^+ transport. This suggests that "membrane stabilization" which in the present context is defined as a block of the Na^+-K^+ leak fluxes, has two effects; one is to slow the cellular leak of K^+ and Na^+ in the ischemic brain, and the other is to reduce ATP consumption and hence oxygen and glucose uptake in normal non-ischemic brain. Lidocaine blocks the Na^+ channels in peripheral nerves, and as will be summarized in this presentation, we have found that this drug in high doses has a similar action in the brain. This membrane-stabilizing effect of lidocaine resembles the effect of hypothermia, and it is evidenced that these two effects are additive. The data leading to these conclusions have been fully accounted for elsewhere (Astrup et al., 1981a; Astrup et al., 1981b), and shall be briefly reviewed here with specific emphasis on prospects of protection of the ischemic brain.

METHODS AND EXPERIMENTAL DESIGN

Dogs were used as experimental animals. In one series the extracellular K^+ concentration in the brain cortex was monitored by a surface potassium electrode (Astrup et al., 1981a), and the effect of thiopental 40 mg/kg, and lidocaine 160 mg/kg on the rate of rise in the surface K^+ concentration studied at brain temperatures of 37, 28, and 18°C, during circulatory arrest. In a second series cerebral blood flow and oxygen and glucose uptake ($CMRO_2$ and CMRgluc) were measured by the sagittal sinus outflow method of Rapela et al. (1967) and Michenfelder et al. (1968). A stepwise experimental procedure was followed. First, the synaptic transmission and associated metabolism was blocked by barbiturate, and second, the assumed high rate of leak fluxes remaining in the functionally inactivated brain with flat EEG was blocked by lidocaine. Studies were carried out at brain temperatures of 37, 28, and 18°C.

In brief, methods included cardiopulmonary by-pass circulation allowing deep hypothermia and well defined circulatory arrest periods and recirculation. Systemic BP was maintained above 50 torr by adjusting the pump speed. Gas flow through the oxygenator was kept constant during cooling allowing arterial pCO_2 to fall with the diminished CO_2 production. Experiments were performed at normoglycemia. Surgical anesthesia was maintained during by-pass circulation by halothane 1% and nitrous oxide 25% in atmospheric air.

RESULTS

Extracellular Potassium Concentration $[K^+]_s$

The increase in the brain surface K^+ concentration $[K^+]_s$, and that indicates the cellular leak of K^+ during circulatory arrest, was unaffected by thiopental 40 mg/kg, but it was slowed by lidocaine 160 mg/kg and hypothermia 28 and 18°C. An additive effect of lidocaine and hypothermia was observed. Figure 1 includes the potassium electrode traces from each single arrest episode in all the experiments, the control condition being halothane-nitrous oxide anesthesia. The rise in $[K^+]_s$ to, for example, 20 mM was reduced from 4-5 min at 37°C and no drugs, to about 30 min at 18°C in combination with lidocaine.

Cerebral Blood Flow and Metabolism

The influence of brain temperature on cerebral metabolism is well described and shall not be further outlined here. We found an Arrhenius type of interrelation according to which log $CMRO_2$ (or CMRgluc) is proportional to °C^{-1}, and described as log $CMRO_2\% = 0.0392 \cdot °C - 0.592$. Q_{10} is then antilog 0.392 = 2.47. These data are in close correspondance with the data published by Michenfelder and Theye (1968).

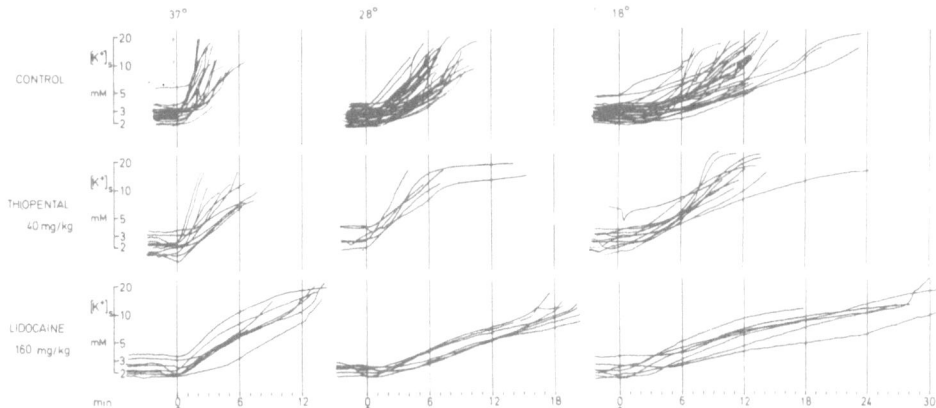

Fig. 1.   Potassium efflux curves grouped according to brain temper-
          ature and drug. The length of the curves indicate circul-
          atory arrest duration, since the recirculation phase is left
          out. (from Astrup et al., <u>Anesthesiology</u>, 55:256, 1981).

     More interest is associated with the effects of pentobarbital
and lidocaine. When studied separately, both drugs caused flat EEG
in the given dose, and this effect was accompanied by profound metabolic depression. In per cent of control, this depression was
equally pronounced at 37, 28 and even at 18°C. When studied in
combination, it was found that lidocaine, when given after pentobarbital (flat EEG), caused additional metabolic depression of about
15-20%, again equally pronounced at the three temperature levels.
On the contrary, when pentobarbital was given after lidocaine (flat
EEG), no additional metabolic depression was observed. The data is
summarized in Table 1.

DISCUSSION

     We interpret the results outlined above in the following way.
Pentobarbital (or thiopental) specificly blocks synaptic transmission
(flat EEG) and inhibits associated energy requiring cell functions,
mainly Na^+-K^+ transport at the synaptic sites, but has no detectable
effect on membrane permeability for these ions and hence no effect on
the Na^+-K^+ leak fluxes or associated ion transport and energy consumption (no slowing of the ischemic K^+ efflux, no additional metabolic depression after lidocaine). Lidocaine has a dual action.
The drug blocks synaptic transmission and associated metabolism (a
"barbiturate-like" effect), and in addition to this the drug causes a
specific block of the Na^+ channels in the membranes (slowing of the
ischemic K^+ efflux, additional metabolic depression after pentobarbital and flat EEG). This is the so-called "membrane stabilizing"

Table 1.   Effect of Pentobarbital and Lidocaine on Cerebral
Oxygen and Glucose Consumption. The Separate
Effects of the Drugs are Shown in Section 1, and
the Combined Effects in Section 2 and Section 3.
Values are Means ± SEM. (From Astrup et al.,
Anesthesiology, 55:263-268, 1981)

| | Section 1 | | | | |
| | CMR_{O_2} Per Cent | | | CMR_{gluc} Per Cent | |
	37°C	28°C	18°C	37°C	28°C
Halothane 1-1.5 Per cent Control	100	100	100	100	100
Pentobarbital (40 mg/kg)					
Mean	69.4	69.6	74.7	74.2	87.2
SEM	5.5	—	—	6.1	—
n	6	3	3	6	3
Lidocaine (160 mg/kg)					
Mean	65.1	71.0	58.0	61.2	73.2
SEM	4.7	—	—	5.1	—
n	6	4	2	6	2
	Section 2				
Pentobarbital (40 mg/kg)	100	100	100	100	100
Lidocaine (160 mg/kg)					
Mean	84.8	84.7	87.7	81.0	72.0
SEM	3.4	—	—	5.3	—
n	6	3	3	6	3
	Section 3				
Lidocaine (160 mg/kg)	100	100	100	100	100
Pentobarbital (40 mg/kg)					
Mean	95.8	104.5	105	101.3	115
SEM	—	—	—	—	—
n	3	2	1	3	2

effect of lidocaine. It should be noted here that lidocaine was
given in a dose sufficiently high to avoid the seizure-eliciting
effect of intermediate doses (Sakabe et al., 1974).

Hypothermia causes progressive flattening of the EEG (a "barbiturate-like" effect), and slowing of the ischemic K^+ efflux (a
"membrane-stabilizing" effect), and these and probably other slowing
effects are associated with profound metabolic depression.

These results in combination with additional studies using
ouabain as an experimental tool to inhibit Na^+-K^+ ATPase and associated Na^+-K^+ transport, have led to the conclusion that total energy
consumption in the brain falls into three categories (Astrup et al.,
1981): one is associated with the intensity of synaptic transmission

and varies with brain work, one is associated with the Na^+-K^+ leak fluxes and its counteracting Na^+-K^+ transport, and the last part is associated with other yet incompletely defined processes such as Ca^{2+} transport, transmitter and protein turnover, axoplasmatic transport and others. This scheme of cerebral energy consumption is outlined in Figure 2, which further indicates the proposed effects of barbiturate, lidocaine and hypothermia as metabolic depressants.

Possible Implications for the Problem of Protection of the Brain during Circulatory Arrest

There is evidence that the irreversible structural ischemic damage, irrespective of its much debated underlying mechanisms, is "uncovered" or "triggered" by the appearance of the ischemic state of membrane failure, i.e., ATP depletion, arrested active transport, net leak fluxes of Na^+, K^+ and Ca^{2+}, and membrane depolarization. The evidence for this mainly comes from the recent discovery of a good concordance between the flow threshold of membrane failure and of infarction development in case of incomplete cerebral ischemia (middle cerebral artery occlusion) (Symon et al., 1975; Astrup et al., 1977; Morawetz et al., 1978; Tamura et al., 1980; Jones et al., 1981). Accordingly, one mode of protection is to prevent if possible, or at least to delay, the ischemic membrane failure as much as possible as indicated by slowing of the ischemic K^+ efflux. In focal ischemia, the ischemic K^+ efflux can be prevented, at least in the acute state, by supporting local blood flow above the critical low threshold below which the active Na^+-K^+ transport fails (Astrup et al., 1981). In complete global ischemia as in circulatory arrest, the ischemic K^+ efflux cannot be prevented, only delayed. Hypothermia and the state of immaturity of the brain represent two conditions of slowed ischemic K^+ efflux, and both these conditions are associated with marked clinical protection against ischemia/hypoxia.

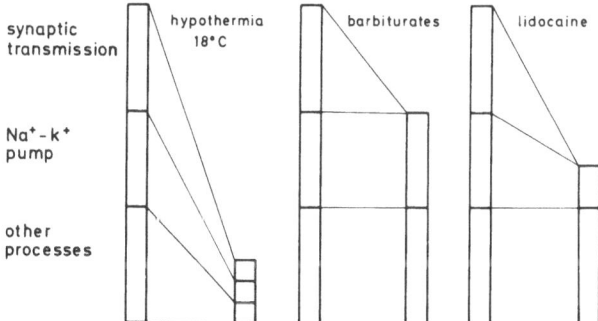

Fig. 2. Schematic presentation of cerebral function and associated metabolism. Inhibition by hypothermia, barbiturates and lidocaine. (See explanation in the text).

This has led to reconsideration of the hypothesis first suggested by
Bures and Buresova (1975), stating that one mode of protection of the
brain during circulatory arrest is a delay of the ischemic membrane
failure. Accordingly, we suggest that lidocaine, which as shown
delays the ischemic membrane failure, induces a similar delay in the
development of irreversible damage, for details see review by Astrup
(1982). It is of interest that the effect of lidocaine seems additive to the effect of hypothermia. This suggests the possibility
of additive protection of this combination. Such a combined effect
may prove useful in selected clinical cases within the fields of
cardiac surgery and neurosurgery requiring prolonged circulatory
arrest during deep hypothermia for the surgical procedure (Dillard et
al., 1971; Silverberg et al., 1981).

REFERENCES

Astrup, J., 1982, Energy-requiring cell functions in the ischemic
        brain, J.Neurosurg., 56:482-497.
Astrup, J., Sørensen, P. Møller., and Sørensen, H. Rahbek, 1981,
        Inhibition of cerebral oxygen and glucose consumption in the
        dog by hypothermia, pentobarbital, and lidocaine,
        Anesthesiology, 55:263-268.
Astrup, J. Siesjö, B. K., and Symon, L., 1981, Thresholds in cerebral
        ischemia - the ischemic penumbra (editorial) Stroke, 8:51-57.
Astrup, J., Skovsted, P., Gjerris, F., and Sørensen, H. Rahbek,
        1981a, Increase in extracellular potassium in the brain during
        circulatory arrest: Effects of hypothermia, lidocaine, and
        thiopental, Anesthesiology, 55:256-262.
Astrup, J., Sørensen, P. M., and Sørensen, H. Rahbek, 1981, Oxygen
        and glucose consumption related to Na-K transport in canine
        brain. Stroke, 12:726-730.
Astrup, J., Symon, L., Branston, N. M., and Lassen, N. A., 1977,
        Cortical evoked potential and extracellular K and H at crit-
        ical levels of brain ischemia, Stroke, 8:51-57.
Bures, J., and Buresova, O., 1957, Die anoxische terminaldepolaris-
        ation als indicator der vulnerabilität der grosshirnrinde bei
        anoxie und ischämie, Pfluegers Arch., 264:325-334.
Dillard, D. H., Mohri, H., and Merendino, K. A., 1971, Correction of
        heart disease in infancy utilizing deep hypothermia and total
        circulatory arrest, J.Thorac.Cardiovasc.Surg., 61:64-69.
Jones, T. H., Morawetz, R. B., Crowell, R. M., 1981, Thresholds of
        focal cerebral ischemia in awake monkeys, J.Neurosurg.,
        54:773-782.
Michenfelder, J. D., Messick, J. M., and Theye, R. A., 1968, Simul-
        taneous cerebral blood flow measured by direct and indirect
        methods, J.Surg.Res., 8:475-481.
Michenfelder, J. D., and Theye, R. A., 1968, Hypothermia: Effect on
        canine brain and whole-body metabolism, Anesthesiology,
        29:1107-1112.

Morawetz, R. B., DeGirolami, U., and Ojemann, R. G., 1978, Cerebral blood flow determined by hydrogen clearance during middle cerebral artery occlusion in unanesthethized monkeys, Stroke, 9:143-149.

Rapela, C. E., Green, H. D., and Denison, A. B., 1967, Baroreceptor reflexes and autoregulation of cerebral blood flow in the dog, Circ.Res., 21:559-568.

Sakabe, T., Maekawa, T., and Ishikawa, T., 1974, The effects of lidocaine on canine cerebral metabolism and circulation related to the electroecephalogram, Anesthesiology, 40:433-441.

Silverberg, G. D., Reitz, B. A., and Ream, A. K., 1981, Hypothermia and cardiac arrest in the treatment of giant aneurysms of the cerebral circulation and hemangioblastoma of the medulla, J.Neurosurg., 55:337-346.

Symon, L., Crockard, H. A., and Dorsch, N. W. C., 1975, Local cerebral blood flow and vascular reactivity in a chronic stable stroke in baboons, Stroke, 6:482-492.

Tamura, A., Asano, T., and Sano, K., 1980, Correlation between rCBF and histological changes following temporal middle cerebral artery occlusion, Stroke, 11:487-493.

BLOOD FLOW AND OXIDATIVE METABOLISM

OF THE YOUNG ADULT AND AGING BRAIN

S. Hoyer

Institut für Pathochemie und Allgemeine
Neurochemie im Zentrum Pathologie der
Universität Heidelberg, Im Neuenheimer Feld 220-221
6900 Heidelberg-1, FRG

During recent decades, an old desire of mankind seems to be
fulfilled: that of becoming older and older. Progress in medical
and social areas has increased the life expectancy of the population,
at least in the highly developed countries. While in West Germany in
1974 about 13% of the population was 65 years and older (Lauter,
1974), this rate increased to about 16% by 1980. The estimated
number of inhabitants aged 65 years and older will still be 16% in
West Germany by the year 2000 although the population will decrease
by 7% (Stat. Bundesamt, 1981). The process of aging is often a
problem of the aging brain. However, physiological or normal cerebral aging should be strictly differentiated from pathological or
abnormal cerebral aging. Different biological aspects will be discussed here in terms of normal cerebral aging to demonstrate similar-
ities and differences in the young adult and aging brain.

In the healthy young adult brain, blood flow is controlled by
cerebral perfusion pressure (CPP) and by the partial pressure of
carbon dioxide in arterial blood ($paCO_2$), respectively. It is well
documented that a reduction of cerebral perfusion pressure by means
of an increased intracranial pressure or by a decreased mean arterial
blood pressure does not seem to change cerebral blood flow over a
wide range of cerebral perfusion pressures from about 50 to 150 mm Hg
(Carlyle and Grayson, 1955; Dinsdale et al.., 1974; Häggendal et al.,
1970; Hamer et al., 1973; Harper, 1966; Hoyer et al., 1974; Johnston
et al., 1972; Jones et al., 1975; Lassen, 1974; Miller et al., 1971,
1972; Miller et al., 1972; Strandgaard et al., 1973; Strandgaard et
al., 1975; Wüllenweber et al., 1967; Zwetnow, 1970). If autoregulation of cerebral blood flow is maintained, no abnormal changes in
oxidative and energy metabolism of the brain were observed within

the range of cerebral perfusion pressure mentioned (Bernsmeier and
Siemons, 1953; Hoyer et al., 1974; Kaasik et al., 1970; Hoyer et al.,
1954; Siesjö et al., 1971; Siesjö and Zwetnow, 1970; Wiedemann et
al., 1979; Zwetnow, 1970) (Table 1).

It is well established that cerebral blood flow changes almost
linearly with $paCO_2$ from about 20 to about 80 mm Hg: it decreases in
hypocapnia and increases in hypercapnia (Alexander et al., 1968;
Alexander et al., 1964; Häggendal and Johansson, 1965; Meyer et al.,
1962; Raichle et al., 1970; Reivich, 1964; Severinghaus and Lassen,
1967; Wollmann et al., 1968). The cerebral metabolic rates of both
oxygen and glucose as well as the energy metabolism of the brain
remain unchanged in both moderate arterial hypo- and hypercapnia
(Alberti et al., 1975; Alexander et al., 1965; Alexander et al.,
1968; Cohen et al., 1968; Cohen et al., 1964; Folbergrova et al.,
1972; Gottstein et al., 1977; Granholm et al., 1969; Granholm and
Siesjö, 1969; Granholm and Siesjö, 1971; Kety and Schmidt, 1946; Kety
and Schmidt, 1948; Wollmann et al., 1965) (Table 2).

In arterial hypoxemia, cerebral blood flow initially increases
slowly but progressively with decreasing arterial partial pressure of
oxygen (paO_2). When paO_2 drops below 55 mm Hg, cerebral blood flow
increases abruptly, indicating a threshold phenomenon. Oxygen consumption was found to remain unchanged until paO_2 had decreased below
25 mm Hg, but both the cerebral uptake of glucose and cerebral release of lactate were enhanced (Cohen et al., 1967; Hamer et al.,
1976; Hamer et al., 1978; Johannsson and Siesjö, 1975; Kety and
Schmidt, 1948; Kogure et al., 1970; McDowall, 1966; Noell and
Schneider, 1942; Shimojyo et al., 1968) (Table 3).

Under physiological conditions, the brain oxidizes only glucose
to obtain energy and thus to meet functional and structural demands
(Gibbs et al., 1942; Gottstein et al., 1963; Hoyer, 1970). Glucose
is transported from arterial blood across the blood-brain barrier
into the brain cells by means of a carrier-facilitated mechanism.
Only 5% of the total amount of glucose used in the brain passes the
blood-brain barrier by diffusion (Bachelard, 1971; Bachelard, 1971;
Bachelard, 1975; Bachelard et al., 1972; Bachelard et al., 1973;
Crone and Thompson, 1970; Nemoto et al., 1978; Oldendorf, 1971;
Oldendorf, 1976; Pardridge and Oldendorf, 1977). In the cytoplasm
of the brain cells, glucose is metabolized glycolytically to pyruvate. The glycolytic flux is mainly regulated by the allosteric
enzyme phosphofructokinase which works in concert with hexokinase
and pyruvate kinase (Newsholme and Start, 1973; Siesjö, 1978).
About 7% of the amount of glucose taken up by the brain is converted
into lactate by means of lactate dehydrogenase and released into the
cerebrovenous blood (Cohen et al., 1967; Erbslöh et al., 1958;
Gottstein et al., 1963; Hoyer, 1970; Siesjö, 1978). In the mitochondria, pyruvate is metabolized by means of the citric acid cycle.
Pyruvate is known to be the substrate for some important biochemical

reactions in the brain (Figure 1). It is the precursor of acetyl-CoA
derived from pyruvate by oxidative decarboxylation by means of pyruvate dehydrogenase (Perry et al., 1980). Acetyl-CoA is a substrate
for the formation of acetylcholine, a most important neurotransmitter
in the brain. However, less than 1% of oxidized pyruvate is converted into acetylcholine. Impairment of pyruvate oxidation, e.g.,
by barbiturates or cyanide, by reducing glucose or oxygen would lead
to proportional impairment of acetylcholine synthesis even if the
impairment is only small (Gibson and Blass, 1976; Gibson et al.,
1975). Pyruvate can be converted into oxaloacetate by means of
pyruvate carboxylase and into malate by means of malate dehydrogenase. These two steps will seem to be obviously used under distinct biochemical conditions to maintain an undisturbed flux through
the glycolytic pathway into the citric acid cycle for oxidation. The
citric acid cycle is extended by a gamma-aminobutyric acid (GABA)
shunt which is connected with an amino acid pool (Sacks, 1957; Sacks,
1965; Sacks, 1969). The breakdown of one mole glucose by complete
aerobic oxidation, i.e., oxidative decarboxylation and oxidative
phosphorylation, thus yields 36 mole ATP (Lehninger, 1971).

It thus becomes clear from many findings mentioned above that
the oxidative metabolism of the healthy young adult brain is normally
characterized by a balance between oxygen and glucose consumption:
under the conditions of moderate arterial hypotension, moderate hypo-
or hypercapnia or moderate arterial hypoxemia, cerebral oxygen consumption is unchanged as compared to resting conditions. However,
cerebral glucose consumption as well as cerebral release of lactate
are found to be increased in moderate arterial hypotension, hypocapnia and hypoxemia, and tend to decrease in hypercapnia (Tables 1,
2 and 3), thus indicating variations in glucose metabolism at the
molecular level.

In moderate arterial hypotension (CPP 71 mmHg), the glucose
concentration in the brain cortex increased significantly but no
further variations of statistical significance could be calculated in
the concentrations of glycolytic, tricarboxylic acid cycle, and high-

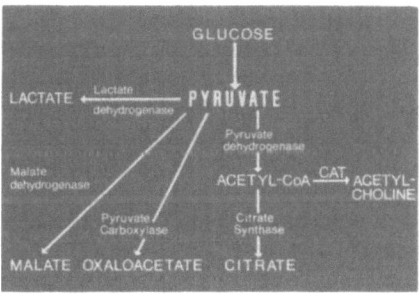

Fig. 1. Metabolism of pyruvate as the precursor of citric acid cycle
         intermediates and acetycholine.

Table 1. Blood Flow and Oxidative Metabolism of the Young Adult in Moderate and Profound Arterial Hypotension

CPP mmHg		CBF ml/100 gmin		CMR-O_2 ml/100 gmin		CMR-GLU mg/100 gmin		CMR-LACT mg/100 gmin		
I	II	I	II	I	II	I	II	I	II	
107	60	54.6	45.7	3.5	3.1					Bernsmeier & Siemons 1953
100	61	51.0	47.0	2.8	3.0					Moyer et. al. 1954
98	71	65.6	64.1	4.2	4.4	4.6	6.2	0.3	1.6	Hoyer et al.
	41		32.2		2.9		3.3		1.1	1974
107	70	60.3	62.1	3.8	4.0	5.2	7.3	0.3	1.3	Wiedemann et al. 1979

Table 2. Blood Flow and Oxidative Metabolism of the Young Adult Brain during Arterial Hypo- and Hypercapnia

paCO_2 mmHg		CBF ml/100 gmin		CMR-O_2 ml/100 gmin		CMR-GLU mg/100 gmin		CMR-LACT mg/100 gmin		
I	II	I	II	I	II	I	II	I	II	
46	28	70	47	4.3	4.9					Kety & Schmidt 1946
43	24	66	41	4.7	4.7					
45	26	52	34	3.5	3.7					Kety & Schmidt 1948
43	52	53	93	3.2	3.3					
37	25	50.8	25.9	2.8	2.7	4.2	4.5	0.5	0.4	Cohen et al., 1964
37	51	50.8	63.8	2.8	2.5	4.2	3.2	0.5	0.6	
41	18	40.5	20.5	2.4	2.5	3.3	3.8	0.3	0.7	Alexander et al., 1965
										Wollman et al., 1965
37	18	61.0	33.9	3.4	3.2	4.6	5.0	0.6	1.1	Alberti et al.,
37	65	61.0	115.7	3.4	3.4	4.6	4.7	0.6	0.5	1975

energy compounds. There is, however, evidence that a moderate activation of the glycolytic flux-controlling enzyme phosphofructokinase may occur, demonstrated by an increase in fructose-1, 6-phosphate concentration. In subcortical white matter, glucose concentration was also elevated to a statistically significant extent, and both glucose-6-phosphate and DHAP were significantly decreased. Lactate concentration increased as compared to control conditions, but the increase fell just short of statistical significance. No activation but rather an inhibition of glycolytic flux might be assumed in subcortical white matter. Glucose metabolism was found to be reduced in cerebral subcortical white matter as compared to brain cortex in both arterial normotension and in moderate arterial hypotension.

Table 3. Blood Flow and Oxidative Metabolism of the Young Adult
          Brain in Moderate and Profound Arterial Hypoxemia

O_2-Vol %		CBF ml/100 gmin		CMR-O_2 ml/100 gmin		CMR-GLU mg/100 gmin		CMR-LACT mg/100 gmin		
I	II	I	II	I	II	I	II	I	II	
18.0.	11.7	54	73	3.4	3.2					Kety & Schmidt 1948
paO_2 mmHg										
89	35	45.0	77.1	3.0	3.1	4.5	5.7	0.2	1.0	Cohen et al., 1967
122	30	58.8	110.9	4.7	4.1	5.2	16.6	0.3	2.3	Hamer et al., 1976
126	45	60.3	84.5	3.8	3.3	5.2	5.9	0.3	1.5	Hamer et al., 1978

Malate, creatine phosphate and ATP decreased significantly to a
similar extent. Lactate, however, was maximally increased only in
moderate arterial hypotension (Hoyer et al., 1983). These changes
agree well with findings of Welsh and Rieder, 1978, who found a 10%
decrease of ATP and a 35-40% decrease of creatine phosphate in subcortical white matter as compared to cortical grey matter, but lactate concentration did not differ between the two tissue compartments
in arterial normotension. In mild cerebral oligemia, Welsh et al.
(1978) demonstrated a decrease in creatine phosphate and ATP and an
increase in lactate concentration in subcortical white matter. It
thus may be concluded that in arterial normotension, normocapnia and
normoxemia, the metabolic state of subcortical white matter is up to
ca. 40% lower than in cortical grey matter. In moderate arterial
hypotension, the metabolic level seems to decrease further, except
for lactate, the concentration of which increased markedly. The
increase in the tissue concentrations of glucose and lactate seems to
be in good agreement with the changes in the cerebral metabolic rates
of glucose and lactate which were both found to be increased in
moderate arterial hypotentsion (see above). There is evidence that
the increase in lactate production occurs only in white matter.

When cerebral perfusion pressure has been reduced below 40 mmHg,
decreases in the concentrations of creatine phosphate and ATP and
increases in ADP, AMP, lactate and pyruvate in brain tissue were
observed (Kaasik et al., 1970; Reulen et al., 1968; Roth et al.,
1967; Siesjö and Zwetnow 1970; Siesjö and Zwetnow 1970) along with
reductions in both oxygen and glucose consumption of the brain (Hamer
et al., 1973; Hoyer et al., 1974).

In arterial hypocapnia, an increased glycolytic flux due to an
activation of the phosphofructokinase step is observed along with a

gradually increasing pool size of citric acid cycle intermediates
with duration of hypocapnia due to a rise in pyruvate concentration
and to enhanced CO_2 fixation at the pyruvate carboxylase step
(Norberg 1976). Excessively low arterial partial pressures of CO_2
below 15 mmHg give rise to additional hypoxic lesions in brain tissue
as demonstrated by a small rise in ADP and a small fall in creatine
phosphate concentrations (MacMillan and Siesjö 1973).

In arterial hypercapnia, the glycolytic flux is inhibited at the
phosphofructokinase step, resulting in a reduced formation of pyruvate although the concentration of glucose increases the more the
hypercapnia increases. Therefore the CO_2 fixation rate is decreased
at the pyruvate carboxylase step yielding to a depletion of citric
acid cycle intermediates. Thus, endogenous brain substrates such as
carbohydrates and amino acids were oxidized instead of glucose when
$paCO_2$ rises further (Borgström et al., 1976; Folbergrova et al.,
1975; Folbegrova et al., 1974; Miller 1975). On the other hand,
cerebral oxygen consumption is found to be unchanged. Increasing
arterial hypercapnia gives rise to a fall in creatine phosphate
concentration in brain tissue, but the energy charge of the adenylate
system remains unchanged even in extreme hypercapnia (Folbergrova et
al., 1972; Folbergrova et al., 1972; Siesjö 1972).

In arterial hypoxemia, the glycolytic flux is obviously increased to maintain energy homeostasis at the onset of tissue hypoxia. As a first reaction of arterial hypoxemia, an activation
of the phosphofructokinase step was found to be responsible for
increased glycolytic flux (Norberg et al., 1975; Norberg and Siesjö
1975). After 30 minutes duration of arterial hypoxemia, the increased glycolytic flux seems to be maintained by activation of the
other flux-controlling steps hexokinase and pyruvate kinase (Hamer
et al., 1978). Since lactacidosis may shift the pH-dependent creatine kinase reaction to maintain ATP stores at the expense of
creatine phosphate, and since some ATP may be formed from increased
glycolysis, no changes could be observed in the concentrations of
adenine nucleotides by decreasing paO_2 to about 25 mmHg (Bachelard et
al., 1974; MacMillan and Siesjö 1973; Norberg and Siesjö 1975; Siesjö
and Nilsson 1971). It may be postulated that the well-established
increase in cerebral blood flow may represent an important homeostatic mechanism under these conditions (Borgström et al., 1975).

In severe arterial hypoxemia with paO_2 below 30 mmHg and ischemia due to carotid clamping (graded oligemia), a decrease in the
cortical concentrations of creatine phosphate, ATP, and energy charge
potential, and an increase in ADP, AMP and lactate could be observed
(Salford 1973). When moderate arterial hypoxemia is associated with
moderate arterial hypotension – a not uncommon situation under clinical conditions – autoregulation of cerebral blood flow has been
found to be abolished and the oxygen consumption of the brain was
reduced (Meyer et al., 1962; Wiedemann et al., 1979). However, the

pool of adenine nucleotides remained unchanged under the conditions
mentioned (Wiedemann et al., 1979).

In healthy non-hospitalized young adult subjects, cerebral blood
flow was measured between 45 and 65 ml/100 g min, CMR-oxygen was
found to be between 3.0 and 3.8 ml/100 g min and CMR-glucose was
measured between 4.5 and 6 mg/100 g min (Cohen et al., 1964;
Gottstein et al., 1963; Hoyer 1970; Kety and Schmidt 1948; Kety and
Schmidt 1948; Mangold et al., 1955; Scheinberg and Stead 1949;
Sokoloff 1966). On the other hand, there are somewhat conflicting
findings in the literature as to whether blood flow and metabolism of
the brain are reduced or are unchanged with advancing age as far as
normal cerebral aging is concerned. Kety (1956) reviewed the results
of several investigations and concluded from them that there is a
remarkable decline in both cerebral blood flow and oxygen uptake from
childhood through adolescence, followed by a more gradual but progressive reduction from the third decade of life onward through middle
and old age. Fazekas et al. (1952) compared mentally healthy people
below and over the age of 50 years. Individuals younger than 50
years did not reveal any variations of blood flow and oxygen consumption of the brain as compared to a group of healthy young volunteers. Individuals over the age of 50 years, however, showed
significant reductions in both brain blood flow and oxygen consumption. It is noteworthy that the individual data of the cerebral
parameters measured scattered very much with age: "normal" values
were found beside reduced ones. Recently Frackowiak et al. (1980)
reported on measurements of cerebral blood flow and the cerebral
metabolic rate of oxygen in both grey and white matter in healthy
volunteers aged from 26 to 74 years. Blood flow and oxygen consumption were found to be reduced in cerebral grey matter with increasing age, but no age-related changes could be observed in cerebral white matters. Similar findings were reported by Naritomi et
al. (1979) with respect to cerebral cortical flow. On the other
hand, Scheinberg et al. (1953) obtained a significantly lower cerebral blood flow in subjects aged from 38 to 79 years with normal
brain functions as compared to a young adult healthy control group,
but CMR-oxygen did not vary between the age groups. Schieve and
Wilson (1953) investigated cerebral blood flow and oxygen consumption
in healthy people at mean ages of 29, 40 and 64 years, respectively.
They did not find any differences in the parameters measured within
these different age groups. The contradiction in these findings
might be due to the fact that young and elderly individuals investigated were both volunteers living in the community and hospitalized
patients. They were designated as "normal" by exclusion of mental or
vascular diseases, but mental normality was not proved by means of
psychological tests, or by EEG or by both. Demonstrating such a
normality by means of several psychometric tests, Lassen et al.
(1960) found a slight but by 99% significantly reduced CMR-oxygen in
mentally normal elderly subjects aged from 66 to 79 years as compared
to healthy young adult controls. In well documented mentally and

physically intact individuals aged 71 years on average, Dastur et al.
(1963) found CMR-oxygen insignificantly decreased by 6%, but CMR-
glucose was decreased significantly by 23% in the healthy elderly.
A similar decrease of CMR-glucose by 26% in elderly healthy subjects
was recently reported by Alavi et al. (1982). Cerebral blood flow
was unchanged in the elderly people investigated by Lassen and Dastur
and their respective colleagues.

It thus becomes evident that cerebral blood flow does not seem
to decline with normal cerebral aging. The small reductions in the
cerebral metabolic rates of oxygen and glucose might tentatively be
accounted for by a progressive but physiological loss of cortical
neurones (Brody 1955), and by the loss of dendrites and dendritic
spines, too (Scheibel 1978; Scheibel 1975). Therefore, cerebral
blood flow would have to be expected to be also decreased. It may,
however, be assumed that the reduction in metabolism due to the nerve
cell loss might give rise to a compensatory increase in cerebral
blood flow so that it appears within the normal range.

The problem as to whether autoregulation of cerebral blood flow
or CO_2 reactivity of the cerebral vessels are unchanged or disturbed
in normal cerebral aging is far from being resolved. No data on
autoregulation of cerebral blood flow in aged normals are available
in the literature. Only scanty results on CO_2 reactivity of cerebral
vessels in normal elderly people are reported. While Schieve and
Wilson (1953) and Dekoninck et al. (1975) described normal responses
of cerebral blood flow to changes in arterial pCO_2, Yamamoto et al.
(1980) found a significant reduction of vasodilatation response to
hypercapnic CO_2 with advancing age.

In experimental animals, London et al. (1981) studied the cerebral glucose utilization during development and aging. They found a
rise in cerebral glucose utilization with development from one to
three months, and a constancy in the following 22 months demonstrating no senescence-associated cerebral changes. Our group investigated the cerebral glucose and energy metabolism in rats being
six or 12 or 24 or 30 months of age which corresponds to 15 or 30 or
60 or 75 years in human life, respectively (Kuhlenbeck 1954). The
glucose concentration in brain cortex was found to be about 1.5 times
higher in 6-month-old animals than in 12-month-old control rats, but
the concentrations did not change between the 12, 24 and 30-month-old
animals. Increases of statistical significance were also found in
fructose-1,6-phosphate, indicating an increased glycolytic flux, as
well as in ATP concentration in 6-month-old animals. In 24 and
30-month-old rats, pyruvate, malate, and creatine phosphate are found
to be reduced, indicating a slight decrease in brain glucose and
energy metabolism with aging (Figure 2) (Ulfert et al., 1982).
Recently, Smith and coworkers (1980) demonstrated in the resting
conscious rat that normal cerebral aging is associated with an in-
homogeneously decreased glucose utilization particularly in auditory

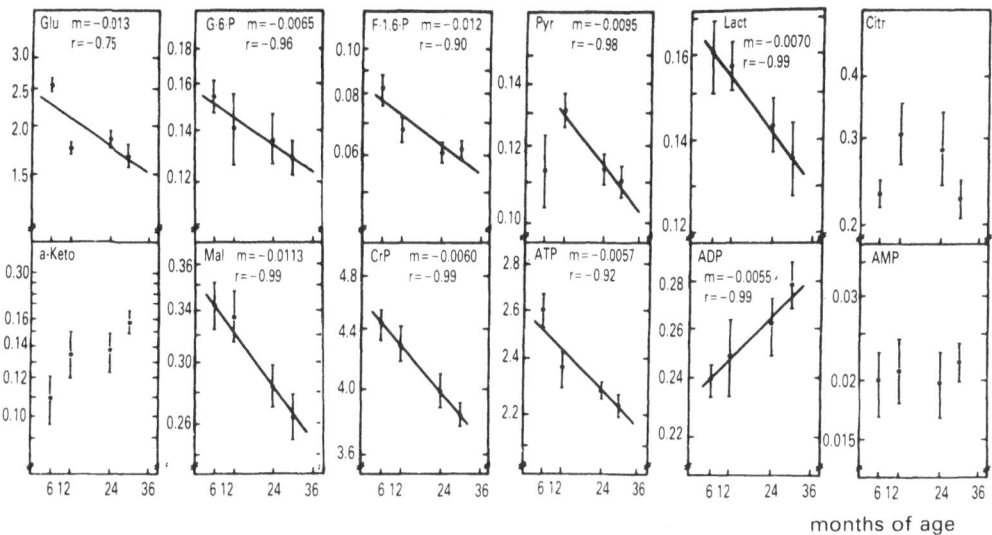

Fig. 2. Semilogarithmical graph of glucose and energy metabolite
concentration (in µmol/g) in brain cortex of rats with
increasing age. The decrease of glucose, fructose-1,6-
phosphate and ATP was statistically significant between
6 and 12 months of age. The concentrations of pyruvate,
malate and creatine phosphate fell statistically significantly between 24 and 30 months of age. Glu: glucose;
G-6-P: glucose-6-phosphate; F-1,6-P: fructose-1,6-phosphate;
Pyr: pyruvate; Lact: lactate; Citr: citrate; α-Keto: α-keto-
glutarate; Mal: malate; CrP: creatine phosphate; ATP:
adenosinetriphosphate; ADP: adenosinediphosphate; AMP:
adenosinemonophosphate.

and visual areas of the brain. The reduction in cerebral glucose
metabolism with aging might be in accordance with the age-dependent
decrease of choline acetyltransferase activity and thus acetylcholine
synthesis as was described by Davies (1979). On the other hand,
Bowen et al. (1979); White et al. (1977) reported on an absence of an
age-dependent decrease of choline acetyltransferase activity in
normal human brains.

     First investigations on the effect of a 15-minute profound
arterial hypoxemia on the glucose and energy metabolism of the aging
brain yielded results which were similar between 2-year-old rats and
1-year-old controls as far as the glycolytic flux is concerned.
The concentrations of creatine phosphate and ATP were found to be
decreased in profound arterial hypoxemia in both age groups. But
profound arterial hypoxemia seems to cause less pronounced changes
in glycolytic flux and citric acid cycle with advancing age obviously
indicating either reduced metabolic demands or reduced homeostatic
capacity or both (Degrell et al., 1981).

It thus seems to be likely that the normally aging brain reacts differently in quantitative terms from the young adult brain. Whether these different reactions on, e.g. arterial hypotension or hypo- and hyperglycemia, etc., would be risks for the aging brain is still unknown. Further investigations are called for.

REFERENCES

Alavi, A., Reivich, M., Ferris, S., Christman, S., Fowler, J., MacGregor, R., Farkas, T., Greenberg, J., Dann, R., and Wolf, A., 1982, Regional cerebral glucose metabolism in aging and senile dementia as determined by 18F-Deoxyglucose and positron emission tomography, Exp.Brain Res., Suppl.5 (in press).

Alberti, E., Hoyer, S., Hamer, J., Stoeckel, H., Packschiess, P., and Weinhardt, F., 1975, The effect of carbon dioxide on cerebral blood flow and cerebral metabolism in dogs, Br.J.Anaesth., 47:941-947.

Alexander, S. C., Cohen, P. J., Wollman, H., Smith, T. C., Reivich, M., and van der Molen, R. A., 1965, Cerebral carbohydrate metabolism during hypocarbia in man. Studies during nitrous oxide anesthesia, Anesthesiology, 26:624-632.

Alexander, S. C., Marshall, B. E., and Agnoli, A., 1968, Cerebral blood flow in the goat with sustained hypocapnia, Scand.J. Clin.Lab.Invest., 22, Suppl.102, VIII C.

Alexander, S. C., Smith, T. C., Strobel, G., Stephen, G. W., and Wollman, H., 1968, Cerebral carbohydrate metabolism of man during respiratory and metabolic alkalosis, J.Appl.Physiol., 24:66-72.

Alexander, S. C., Wollman, H., Cohen, P. J., and Behar, M., 1964, Cerebrovascular response to $paCO_2$ during halothane anesthesia in man, J.Appl.Physiol., 19:561-565.

Bachelard, H. S., 1971, Specificity and kinetic properties of mono-saccharide uptake into guinea pig cerebral cortex in vitro, J.Neurochem., 13:213-222.

Bachelard, H. S., 1971, Glucose transport and phosphorylation in the control of carbohydrate metabolism in the brain, in: "Brain Hypoxia," J. B. Brierly and B. S. Meldrum, eds., Heinemann, London.

Bachelard, H. S., 1975, How does glucose enter brain cells? in: "Brain Work. The Coupling of Function, Metabolism and Blood Flow in the Brain," D. H. Ingvar and N. A. Lassen, eds., Munksgaard, Copenhagen.

Bachelard, H. S., Daniel, P. M., Love, E. R., and Pratt, O. E., 1972, The in vivo influx of glucose into the brain of the rat compared with the net cerebral uptake, J.Physiol.(London), 222:149-150P.

Bachelard, H. S., Daniel, P. M., Love, E. R., and Pratt, O. E., 1973, The transport of glucose into the brain of the rat in vivo, Proc.Roy.Soc.B., 183:71-82.

Bachelard, H. S., Lewis, L. D., Ponten, U., and Siesjö, B. K., 1974, Mechanisms activating glycolysis in the brain in arterial hypoxia, J.Neurochem., 22:395-401.

Bernsmeier, A., and Siemons, K., 1953, Der Hirnkreislauf bei der gesteuerten experimentellen Hypotension (Hypotension controllée), Schweiz.Med.Wschr., 83:210-212.

Borgström, L., Johannsson, H., and Siesjö, B. K., 1975, The relationship between arterial pO_2 and cerebral blood flow in hypoxic hypoxia, Acta Physiol.Scand., 93:423-432.

Borgström, L., Norberg, K., and Siesjö, B. K., 1976, Glucose consumption in rat cerebral cortex in normoxia, hypoxia and hypercapnia, Acta Physiol.Scand., 96:569-574.

Bowen, D. M., White, P., Spillane, J. A., Goodhardt, M. J., Curzon, G., Jwangoff, P., Meier-Ruge, W., and Davison, A. N., 1979, Accelerated ageing or selective neuronal loss as an important cause of dementia? Lancet I, 11-14.

Brody, H., 1955, Organization of cerebral cortex. III. A study of aging in human cerebral cortex, J.Comp.Neurol., 102:511-556.

Carlyle A., and Grayson, J., 1955, Blood pressure and the regulation of brain blood flow, J.Physiol.(London), 127:15-16P.

Cohen, P. J., Alexander, S. C., Smith, T. C., Reivich, M., and Wollman, H., 1967, Effects of hypoxia and normocarbia on cerebral blood flow and metabolism in conscious man, J.Appl.Physiol., 23:183-189.

Cohen, P. J., Alexander, S. C., and Wollman, H., 1968, Effects of hypocarbia and of hypoxia with normocarbia on cerebral blood flow and metabolism in man, Scand.J.Clin.Lab.Invest., 22, Suppl.102, IV A.

Cohen, P. J., Wollman, H., Alexander, S. C., Chase, P. E., and Behar, M. G., 1964, Cerebral carbohydrate metabolism in man during halothane anesthesia. Effects of $paCO_2$ on some aspects of carbohydrate utilization, Anesthesiology, 25:185-191.

Crone, C., and Thompson, A. M., 1970, Permeability of brain capillaries, in: "Capillary Permeability," C. Crone and N. A. Lassen, eds., Munskgaard, Copenhagen.

Dastur, D. K., Lane, M. H., Hansen, D. B., Kety, S. S., Butler, R. N., Perlin, S., and Sokoloff, L., 1963, Effects of aging on cerebral circulation and metabolism in man, in: "Human Aging. A Biological and Behavioral Study," J. E. Birren, R. N. Butler, S. W. Greenhouse, L. Sokoloff, and M. R. Yarrow, eds., US Govt. Print. Off., Washington, D.C.

Davies, P., 1979, Neurotransmitter-related enzymes in senile dementia of the Alzheimer type, Brain Res., 171:319-327.

Degrell, I., Krier, C., and Hoyer, S., 1981, Carbohydrate and energy metabolism of the aging rat brain in severe arterial hypoxemia, in: "Brain Aging". 2nd Int.Ernst Reuter Symp. Berlin.

Dekoninck, W. J., Collard, M., and Jacquy, J., 1975, Comparative study of cerebral vasoactivity in vascular sclerosis of the brain in elderly men, Stroke., 6:673-677.

Dinsdale, H. B., Robertson, D. M., and Haas, R. A., 1974, Cerebral blood flow in acute hypertension, Arch.Neurol., 31:80-87.

Erbslöh, F., Klärner, P., and Bernsmeier, A., 1958, Die Milchsäureab-
    gabe des menschlichen Gehirns, Pflügers Arch.ges.Physiol.,
    268:120-133.
Fazekas, J. F., Alman, R. W., and A. N. Bessman, 1952, Cerebral
    physiology of the aged, Am.J.Med.Sci., 223:245-257.
Folbergrova, J., MacMillan, V., and Siesjö, B. K., 1972, The effect
    of moderate and marked hypercapnia upon the energy state and
    upon the cytoplasmatic NADH/NAD$^+$-ratio of the rat brain,
    J.Neurochem., 19:2497-2505.
Folbergrova, J., MacMillan, V., and Siesjö, B. K., 1972, The effect
    of hypercapnic acidosis upon some glycolytic and Krebs cycle-
    associated intermediates in the rat brain, J.Neurochem.,
    19:2507-2517.
Folbergrova, J., Norberg, K., Quistorff, B., and Siesjö, B. K., 1975,
    Carbohydrate and amino acid metabolism in rat cerebral cortex
    in moderate and extreme hypercapnia, J.Neurochem., 25:457-462.
Folbergrova, J., Ponten, U., and Siesjö, B. K., 1974, Patterns of
    changes in brain carbohydrate metabolites, amino acids and
    organic phosphates at increased carbon dioxide tensions,
    J.Neurochem., 22:1115-1125.
Frackowiak, R. S. J., Lenzi, G. L., Jones, T., and Heather, J. D.,
    1980, Quantitative measurements of regional cerebral blood
    flow and oxygen metabolism in man using ^{15}O and positron
    emission tomography: Theory, procedure and normal values,
    J.Comput.Assist.Tomogr., 4:727-736.
Gibbs, E. L., Lennox, W. G., Nims, L. F., and Gibbs, F. A., 1942,
    Arterial and cerebral venous blood. Arterial-venous dif-
    ferences in man, J.Biol.Chem., 144:325-332.
Gibson, G. E., and Blass, J. P., 1976, Impaired synthesis of
    acetylcholine in brain accompanying hypoglycemia and mild
    hypoxia, J.Neurochem., 27:37-42.
Gibson, G. E., Jope, R., and Blass, J. P., 1975, Reduced synthesis of
    acetylcholine accompanying impaired oxidation of pyruvic acid
    in rat brain minces, Biochem.J., 148:17-29.
Gottstein, U., Bernsmeier, A., and Sedlmeyer, I., 1963, Der Kohlen-
    hydratstoffwechsel des menschlichen Gehirns. I. Untersuchungen
    mit substratspezifischen enzymatischen Methoden bei normaler
    Hirndurchblutung, Klin.Wschr., 41:943-948.
Gottstein, U., Gabriel, F. H., Held, K., and Textor, Th., 1977,
    Continuous monitoring of arterial and cerebral venous glucose
    concentrations in man. Advantage, procedure and results, in:
    "Blood Glucose Monitoring. Methodology and Clinical Ap-
    plication of Continuous in vivo Glucose Analysis," Thieme,
    Stuttgart.
Granholm, L., Lukjanova, L., and Siesjö, B. K., 1969, The effect of
    marked hyperventilation upon tissue levels of NADH, lactate,
    pyruvate, phosphocreatine and adenosine phosphates of rat
    brain, Acta Physiol.Scand., 77:179-199.
Granholm, L., and Siesjö, B. K., 1969, The effects of hypercapnia and
    hypocapnia upon the cerebrospinal fluid lactate and pyruvate

concentrations and upon the lactate, pyruvate, ATP, ADP,
phosphocreatine and creatine concentrations of cat brain
tissue, Acta Physiol.Scand., 75:257-266.

Granholm, L., and Siesjö, B. K., 1971, The effect of combined
respiratory and non-respiratory alkalosis on energy
metabolites and acid-base parameters in rat brain,
Acta Physiol.Scand., 81:307-314.

Häggendal, E., 1965, Blood flow autoregulation of the cerebral grey
matter with comments on its mechanism, Acta Neurol.Scand., 41:
Suppl.14, 104-110.

Häggendal, E., and Johansson, B., 1965, Effects of arterial carbon
dioxide tension and oxygen saturation on cerebral blood flow
autoregulation in dogs, Acta Physiol.Scand., 66:Suppl.258,
27-53.

Häggendal, E., Löfgren, J., Nilsson, N. J., and Zwetnow, N. N., 1970,
Effects of varied cerebrospinal fluid pressure on cerebral
blood flow in dogs, Acta Physiol.Scand., 79:262-271.

Hamer, J., Hoyer, S., Alberti, E., and Weinhardt, F., 1976, Cerebral
blood flow and oxidative brain metabolism during and after
moderate and profound arterial hypoxaemia, Acta Neurochir.,
33:141-150.

Hamer, J., Hoyer, S., Stoeckel, H., Alberti, E., and Weinhardt, F.,
1973, Cerebral blood flow and cerebral metabolism in acute
increase of intracranial pressure, Acta Neurochir., 28:95-110.

Hamer, J., Wiedemann, K., Berlet, H., Weinhardt, F., and Hoyer, S.,
1978, Cerebral glucose and energy metabolism, cerebral oxygen
consumption and blood flow in arterial hypoxaemia,
Acta Neurochir., 44:151-160.

Harper, A. M., 1966, Autoregulation of cerebral blood flow: Influence
of the arterial blood pressure on the blood flow through the
cerebral cortex, J.Neurol.Neurosurg.Psychiat., 29:398-403.

Hoyer, S., 1970, Der Aminosäurenstoffwechsel des normalen mensch-
lichen Gehirns, Klin.Wschr., 48:1239-1243.

Hoyer, S., Hamer, J., Alberti, E., Stoeckel, H., and Weinhardt, F.,
1974, The effect of stepwise arterial hypotension on blood
flow and oxidative metabolism of the brain, Pflügers
Arch.ges.Physiol., 351:161-172.

Hoyer, S., Wiedemann, K., Krier, C., and Degrell, I., Effect of
moderate arterial hypotension on glucose and energy metabolism
in cerebral grey and subcortical white matter in dogs (in
preparation).

Johannson, H., and Siesjö, B. K., 1975, Cerebral blood flow and
oxygen consumption in the rat in hypoxic hypoxia,
Acta Physiol.Scand., 93:269-276.

Johnston, I. H., Rowan, J. O., Harper, A. M., Jennett, W. B., 1972,
Raised intracranial pressure and cerebral blood flow. Cisterna
magna infusion in primates, J.Neurol.Neurosurg.Psychiat.,
35:285-296.

Jones, J. V., Strandgaard, S., MacKenzie, E. T., Fitch, W., Lawrie,
T. D. V., and Harper, A. M., 1975, Autoregulation of cerebral

blood flow in chronic hypertension, in: "Blood Flow and
  Metabolism in the Brain," A. M. Harper, W. B. Jennett, J. D.
  Miller, and J. O. Rowan, eds., Churchill Livingstone,
  Edinburgh - London - New York.
Kaasik, A. E., Nilsson, L., and Siesjö, B. K., 1970, The effect of
  arterial hypotension upon the lactate, pyruvate and bicarb-
  onate concentrations of the brain tissue and cisternal CSF and
  upon the tissue concentrations of phosphocreatine and adenine
  nucleotides in anesthetized rats, Acta Physiol.Scand.,
  78:448-458.
Kety, S. S., 1956, Human cerebral blood flow and oxygen consumption
  as related to aging, J.Chron.Dis., 3:478-486.
Kety, S. S., and Schmidt, C. F., 1946, The effects of active and
  passive hyperventilation on cerebral blood flow, cerebral
  oxygen consumption, cardiac output and blood pressure of
  normal young men, J.Clin.Invest., 25:107-119.
Kety, S. S., and Schmidt, C. F., 1948, The nitrous oxide method for
  the quantitative determination of cerebral blood flow in man:
  Theory, procedure and normal values, J.Clin.Invest.,
  27:476-483.
Kety, S. S., and Schmidt, C. F., 1948, The effects of altered
  arterial tensions of carbon dioxide and oxygen on cerebral
  blood flow and cerebral oxygen consumption of normal young
  men, J.Clin.Invest., 27:484-492.
Kogure, K., Scheinberg, P., Reinmuth, O. M., Fujishima, M., and
  Busto, R., 1970, Mechanisms of cerebral vasodilation in
  hypoxia, J.Appl.Physiol., 29:223-229.
Kuhlenbeck, H., 1954, Some histological age changes in the rat's
  brain and their relationship to comparable changes in the
  human brain, Confin.Neurol., 14:329-342.
Lassen, N. A., 1974, Control of cerebral circulation in health and
  disease, Circulation Res., 34:749-760.
Lassen, N. A., Feinberg, I., and Lane, M. H., 1960, Bilateral studies
  of cerebral oxygen uptake in young and aged normal subjects
  and in patients with organic dementia, J.Clin.Invest.,
  39:491-500.
Lauter, H., 1974, Epidemiologische Aspekte alterspsychiatrischer
  Erkrankungen, Nervenarzt, 45:277-288.
Lehninger, A. L., 1971, Bioenergetik. Molekulare Grundlagen der
  biologischen Energieumwandlungen, Thieme, Stuttgart.
London, E. D., Nespor, S. M., Ohata, M., and Rapoport, S. I., 1981,
  Local cerebral glucose utilization during development and
  aging of the Fischer-344 rat, J.Neurochem., 37:217-221.
MacDowall, D. G., 1966, Interrelationship between blood oxygen
  tension and cerebral blood flow, in: "Oxygen Measurements in
  Blood and Tissues," J. D. Payne and D. W. Hill, ed., Churchill
  Livingston, London.
MacMillan, V., and Siesjö, B. K., 1972, Brain energy metabolism in
  hypoxemia, Scand.J.Clin.Lab.Invest., 30:126-136.

MacMillan, V., and Siesjö, B. K., 1973, The influence of hypocapnia upon intracellular pH and upon some carbohydrate substrates, amino acids and organic phosphates in the brain, J.Neurochem., 21:1283-1299.

Mangold, R., Sokoloff, L., Therman, P. O., Conner, E. H., Kleinermann, J. I., and Kety, S. S., 1955, The effects of sleep and lack of sleep on the cerebral circulation and metabolism of normal young men, J.Clin.Invest., 34:1092-1100.

Meyer, J. S., Gotoh, F., Tazaki, Y., Hamaguchi, K., Ishikawa, S., Novailhat, F., and Symon, L., 1962, Regional cerebral blood flow and metabolism in vivo. Effects of anoxia, hyperglycemia, ischemia, acidosis, alkalosis and alterations of blood pCO_2, Arch.Neurol., 7:560-581.

Miller, A. L., Hawkins, R. A., and Veech, R. L., 1975, Decreased rate of glucose utilization by rat brain in vivo after exposure to atmospheres containing high concentrations of CO_2, J.Neurochem., 25:553-558.

Miller, J. D., Stanek, A. E., and Langfitt, T. W., 1971/72, A comparison of autoregulation to changes in intracranial and arterial pressure in the same preparation, Europ.Neurol., 6:34-38.

Miller, J. D., Stanek, A., and Langfitt, T. W., 1972, Concepts of cerebral perfusion pressure and vascular compression during intracranial hypertension, Progr.Brain Res., 35:411-432.

Moyer, J. H., Morris, G., and Smith, C. P., 1954, Cerebral hemodynamics during controlled hypotension induced by the continuous infusion of ganglionic blocking agents, J.Clin.Invest., 33:1081-1088.

Naritomi, H., Meyer, J. S., Sakai, F., Yamaguchi, F., and Shaw, T., 1979, Effects of advancing age on regional cerebral blood flow. Studies in normal subjects and subjects with risk factors for atherothrombotic stroke, Arch.Neurol., 36:410-416.

Nemoto, E. M., Stezoski, S. W., and MacMurdo, D., 1978, Glucose transport across the rat blood-brain barrier during anesthesia, Anesthesiology, 49:170-176.

Newsholme, E. A., and Start, C., 1973, "Regulation in Metabolism," Wiley, Chichester - New York - Brisbane - Toronto.

Noell, W., and Schneider, M., 1942, Über die Durchblutung und die Sauerstoffversorgung des Gehirns. I. Die Gehirndurchblutung, Pflügers Arch.ges.Physiol., 246:181-249.

Norberg, K., 1976, Changes in cerebral metabolism induced by hyperventilation at different blood glucose levels, J.Neurochem., 26:353-359.

Norberg, K., Quistorff, B., and Siesjö, B. K., 1975, Effects of hypoxia of 10-45 seconds duration on energy metabolism on the cerebral cortex of unanaesthetized and anaesthetized rats, Acta Physiol.Scand., 95:301-310.

Norberg, K., and Siesjö, B. K., 1975, Cerebral metabolism in hypoxic hypoxia. I. Pattern of activation of glycolysis, a re-evaluation, Brain Res., 86:31-44.

Norberg, K., and Siesjö, B. K., 1975, Cerebral metabolism in hypoxic hypoxia. II. Citric acid cycle intermediates and associated amino acids, Brain Res., 86:45-54.

Oldendorf, W. H., 1971, Brain uptake of radiolabeled amino acids, amines and hexoses after arterial injection, Am.J.Physiol., 221:1629-1639.

Oldendorf, W. H., 1976, Blood-brain barrier, in: "Brain Metabolism and Cerebral Disorders," H. E. Himwich, ed., Spectrum, New York.

Pardridge, W. M., and Oldendorf, W. H., 1977, Transport of metabolic substrates through the blood-brain barrier, J.Neurochem., 28:5-12.

Perry, E. K., Perry, R. H., Tomlinson, B. E., Blessed, G., and Gibson, P. H., 1980, Coenzyme A acetylating enzymes in Alzheimer's disease: Possible cholinergic "compartment" of pyruvate dehydrogenase, Neurosci.Lett., 18:105-110.

Raichle, M. E., Posner, J. B., and Plum, F., 1970, CBF during and after hyperventilation, Arch.Neurol., 23:394-403.

Reivich, M., 1964, Arterial pCO_2 and cerebral hemodynamics, Am.J.Physiol., 206:25-35.

Reulen, H. J., Steude, U., Brendel, W., and Medzihradsky, F., 1968, Elektrolyt-und Metabolitkonzentrationen im Gehirn nach normovolämische Drucksenkung, Z.ges.Exp.Med., 146:241-260.

Roth, E., Schüler, W., Suleder, O., and Sobol, B., 1967, Metabolit-konzentrationen in Herz, Gehirn, Niere und Leber des Hundes bei kontrollierter Hypotension, Z.ges.Exp.Med., 144:258-272.

Sacks, W., 1957, Cerebral metabolism of isotopic glucose in normal human subjects, J.Appl.Physiol., 10:37-44.

Sacks, W., 1965, Cerebral metabolism of doubly labeled glucose in humans in vivo, J.Appl.Physiol., 20:117-130.

Sacks, W., 1969, Cerebral metabolism in vivo, in: "Handbook of Neurochemistry, Vol.1," A. Lajtha, ed., Plenum, New York.

Salford, L. G., Plum, F., and Siesjö, B. K., 1973, Graded hypoxia-oligemia in rat brain. I. Biochemical alterations and their implications, Arch.Neurol., 29:227-233.

Scheibel, A. B., 1978, Structural aspects of the aging brain: Spine systems and the dendritic arbor, in: "Alzheimer's Disease: Senile Dementia and Related Disorders (Aging Vo.7)," R. Katzman, R. D. Terry, and K. L. Bick, eds., Raven, New York.

Scheibel, M. E., Lindsay, R. D., Tomiyasu, U., and Scheibel, A. B., 1975, Progressive dendritic changes in aging human cortex, Exp.Neurol., 47:392-403.

Scheinberg, P., Blackburn, I., Rich, M., and Saslaw, M., 1953, Effects of aging on cerebral circulation and metabolism, Arch.Neurol.Psychiat., 70:77-85.

Scheinberg, P., and Stead, jr., E. A., 1949, The cerebral blood flow in male subjects as measured by the nitrous oxide technique: Normal values for blood flow, oxygen utilization, glucose utilization and peripheral resistance with observations on the effect of tilting and anxiety, J.Clin.Invest., 28:1163-1171.

Schieve, J. F., and Wilson, W. P., 1953, The influence of age, anesthesia and cerebral arteriosclerosis on cerebral vascular activity to CO_2, Am.J.Med., 15:171-174.

Severinghaus, J. W., and Lassen, N. A., 1967, Step hypocapnia to separate arterial from tissue pCO_2 in the regulation of cerebral blood flow, Circulation Res., 20:272-278.

Shimojyo, S., Scheinberg, P., Kogure, K., and Reinmuth, O. M., 1968, The effects of graded hypoxia upon transient cerebral blood flow and oxygen consumption, Neurology(Minneap.) 18:127-133.

Siesjö, B. K., 1978, "Brain Energy Metabolism," Wiley, Chichester - New York - Brisbane - Toronto.

Siesjö, B. K., Folbergrova, J., and MacMillan, V., 1972, The effect of hypercapnia upon intracellular pH in the brain, evaluated by the bicarbonate-carbonic acid method and from the creatine phosphokinase equilibrium, J.Neurochem., 19:2483-2495.

Siesjö, B. K., and Nilsson, L., 1971, The influence of arterial hypoxemia upon labile phosphates and upon extracellular and intracellular lactate and pyruvate concentrations in the rat brain, Scand.J.Clin.Lab.Invest., 27:83-96.

Siesjö, B. K., Nilsson, L., Rokeach, M., and Zwetnow, N. N., 1971, Energy metabolism of the brain at reduced cerebral perfusion pressures and in arterial hypoxaemia, in: "Brain Hypoxia," J. B. Brierley and B. S. Meldrum, eds., Heinemann, London.

Siesjö, B. K., and Zwetnow, N. N., 1970, Effects of increased cerebrospinal fluid pressure upon adenine nucleotides and upon lactate and pyruvate in the rat brain, Acta Neurol.Scand., 46:187-202.

Siesjö, B. K., and Zwetnow, N. N., 1970, The effect of hypovolemic hypotension on extra- and intracellular acid-base parameters and energy metabolism in the rat brain, Acta Physiol.Scand., 79:114-124.

Smith, C. B., Goochee, C., Rapoport, I., and Sokoloff, L., 1980, Effects of ageing on local rates of cerebral glucose utilization in the rat, Brain, 103:351-365.

Sokoloff, L., 1966, Cerebral circulatory and metabolic changes associated with aging, Res.Pub.Ass.Nerv.Ment.Dis., 41:237-254.

Statistisches Bundesamt FRG (1981).

Strandgaard, S., Mackenzie, E. T., Sengupta, D., Rowan, J. O., Lassen, N. A., and Harper, A. M., 1974, Upper limit of autoregulation of cerebral blood flow in the baboon, Circulation Res., 34:435-440.

Strandgaard, S., Olesen, J., Skinhøj, E., and Lassen, N. A., 1973, Autoregulation of brain circulation in severe arterial hypertension, Br.Med.J., 1:507-510.

Strandgaard, S., Sengupta, D., Mackenzie, E. T., Rowan, J. O., Olesen, J., Skinhøj, E., Lassen, N. A., and Harper, A. M., 1975, The lower and upper limits for autoregulation of cerebral blood flow, in: "Cerebral Circulation and Metabolism," T. W. Langfitt, L. C. McHenry, jr., M. Reivich, and H. Wollman, eds., Springer, New York, Heidelberg, Berlin.

Ulfert, G., Schmidt, U., and Hoyer, S., 1982, Glucose and energy
    metabolism of rat cerebral cortex during aging, Exp.Brain
    Res., Suppl.5 (in press).
Welsh, F. A., O'Connor, M. J., and Marcy, V. R., 1978, Effect of
    oligemia on regional metabolite levels in cat brain,
    J.Neurochem., 31:311-319.
Welsh, F. A., Rieder, W., 1978, Evaluation of in situ freezing of cat
    brain by NADH fluorescence, J.Neurochem., 31:299-309.
White, P., Hiley, C. R., Goodhardt, M. J., Carrasco, L. H., Keet, J.
    P., Williams, J. E. J., and Bowen, D. M., 1977, Neocortical
    cholinergic neurons in elderly people, Lancet II, 668-671.
Wiedemann, K., Weinhardt, F., Hamer, J., Wund, G., Berlet, H., and
    Hoyer, S., 1979, Einfluß von gleichzeitiger mäßiger arteriel-
    ler Hypoxamie und mäßiger hypovolämischer Hypotension auf
    Gehirndurchblutung, oxidativen und Energiestoffwechsel des
    Gehirns beim Hund, Anaesthesist, 28:290-298.
Wollman, H., Alexander, S. C., Cohen, P. J., Smith, T. C., Chase, P.
    E., and van der Molen, R. A., 1965, Cerebral circulation
    during anesthesia and hyperventilation in man. Thiopental
    induction to nitrous oxide and d-tubocurarine, Anesthesiology,
    26:329-334.
Wollman, H., Smith, T. C., Stephen, G. W., Colton, E. T., Gleaton, H.
    E., and Alexander, S. C., 1968, Effects of extremes of respir-
    atory and metabolic alkalosis on cerebral blood flow in man,
    J.Appl.Physiol., 24:60-65.
Wüllenweber, R., Gött, U., and Szántó, J., 1967, Beobachtungen zur
    Regulation der Hirndurchblutung, Acta Neurochir., 16:137-153.
Yamamoto, M., Meyer, J. S., Sakai, F., and Yamaguchi, F., 1980, Aging
    and cerebral vasodilator responses to hypercarbia. Responses
    in normal aging and in persons with risk factors for stroke,
    Arch.Neurol., 37:489-496.
Zwetnow, N. N., 1970, Effects of increased cerebrospinal fluid
    pressure on the blood flow and on the energy metabolism of
    the brain, Acta Physiol.Scand.Suppl., 339:1-31.
Zwetnow, N. N., 1970, The influence of an increased intracranial
    pressure on the lactate, pyruvate, bicarbonate, phospho-
    creatine, ATP, ADP and AMP concentrations of the cerebral
    cortex of dogs, Acta Physiol.Scand., 79:158-166.

III

CEREBRAL ELECTRICAL ACTIVITY DURING SYSTEMIC HYPOTENSION IN NEUROANESTHESIA

ELECTRICAL MONITORING OF THE BRAIN IN INDUCED HYPOTENSION

AN INTRODUCTION TO THE SESSION

D. G. McDowall

Department of Anaesthesia
The University of Leeds
England

The proportion of slow-wave activity in the EEG increases in profound hypotension and then burst suppression appears. The duration of the isoelectric periods increases in length and if the blood pressure (BP) is low enough, the record finally becomes isoelectric.

In a study of drug-induced hypotension, Morris and colleagues (1982) have shown that major depression of the EEG occurs at higher values of cerebral cortical blood flow than those at which K^+ is released into the extracellular fluid (ecf) of the cerebral cortex of the cat. This observation conforms to the penumbra concept of Astrup and colleagues (1977) which, however, was based on measurement of sensory evoked potentials in focal cerebral ischaemia.

There is a time dimension involved in addition. In the experiments of Morris et al. (1982) if an animal was held at a given reduced BP for some 30 min, EEG deterioration was sometimes delayed by 15-20 min. It is not clear whether this delayed deterioration in the EEG is due to failing cerebral perfusion during prolonged hypotension or whether it is due to an accumulation of the total ischaemic insult time at low BP due, for example, to neurotransmitter depletion.

The relationship of electrical depression to ischaemic cell damage is not fully elucidated. However, Brierley and colleagues (1980) found in an animal experimental study, that an isoelectric EEG always preceded ischaemic cell damage and Malone, Prior and Scholtz (1981) in a neuropathological examination of the brains of patients dying after cardiac surgery, demonstrated that depression of electrical activity had always been present for not less than 7 min in patients whose brains subsequently showed ischaemic cell damage.

It would therefore appear from the penumbra flow concept and the neuropathological evidence, that monitoring of the brain's electrical activity will always give warning of severe cerebral cortical ischaemia. Once significant EEG changes appear the margins of flow, blood pressure and time are narrow and, in my view, should not be exploited clinically, i.e., the appearance of major EEG changes during induced hypotension is an indication to raise the BP immediately.

Monitoring of the EEG in the hostile electrical environment of an operating theatre is probably not practicable as a routine. Furthermore, the necessary expertise in EEG interpretation will often not be available. As a consequence, many have looked for alternative methods of displaying the information. The cerebral function monitor (cfm) (Maynard et al., 1969) is one such approach which has been used successfully in cardiac surgery, carotid artery surgery and induced hypotension (Prior, 1979; Patel, 1981). The record is reasonably free of electrical artefacts and is very easy to interpret. It may lack sensitivity in detecting the earliest changes, since separation of electrical activity into frequency bands is not performed, but this feature has been added in the advanced cfm which is shortly to be made available. One further limitation is that only one bipolar signal is handled by the instrument, so that the electrical activity shown refers only to two areas of cortex under the recording electrodes. This is probably not too severe a disadvantage during global ischaemia produced by hypotension. It might be so, however, in a patient with an abnormal arterial inflow tree, since this might shift the ischaemic areas away from the boundary zones over which the cfm electrodes are normally positioned.

Ishikawa and I (1981) have used the cfm in an experimental study of induced hypotension and were able to show that severe electrical depression occurred earlier during trimetaphan (TMP) than during nitroprusside (NTP) hypotension at the same low BP.

Other approaches used in the routine clinical monitoring of brain electrical activity have included compressed spectral array and various ratios of electrical activity in different frequency bands. None of these has achieved the levels of acceptance of the cfm in the United Kingdom.

Sensory evoked potentials have been used but, as Prior will discuss in the Symposium, these monitor only certain neuronal circuits which may not be the most sensitive to hypotension-induced ischaemia. Timing the evoked response transit from the upper cervical spine to the sensory cortex is a modification of the technique which avoids the complication introduced by variation in the peripheral nerve conduction time (Hume & Cant, 1978; Symon et al., 1979).

Finally, the directly evoked cortical potential has been used with both stimulating and recording electrodes placed directly on the

exposed cortex. Eisenberg and colleagues (1979) have monitored
induced hypotension during neurosurgery with this technique, but of
course it only gives information for the relatively small area of
cortex on which the electrodes are placed. None the less, in the
experience of Jones and colleagues (1979), the post-operative problems of induced hypotension in neurosurgery usually occur in the
territory of the operation and result from a combination of hypotension and vasospasm, or vessel clipping. In neurosurgery, therefore, the critical area for EEG monitoring may be the exposed area of
cortex.

REFERENCES

Astrup, J., Symon, L., Branston, N. M., and Lassen, N. A., 1977,
        Cortical evoked potential and extracellular K^+ and H^+ at
        critical levels of brain ischemia, Stroke, 8:51-57.
Brierley, J. B., Prior, P. F., Calverley, J., Jackson, S. J., and
        Brown, A. W., 1980, The pathogenesis of ischaemic neuronal
        damage along the cerebral arterial boundary zones in papio
        anubis. Brain, 103:929-965.
Eisenberg, H. M., Turner, J. W., Teasdale, G., Rowan, J., Feinstein,
        R., and Grossman, R. E., 1979, Monitoring of cortical excita-
        bility during induced hypotension in aneurysm operations,
        J.Neurosurg., 50:595-602.
Hume, A. L., and Cant, B. R., 1978, Conduction time in central
        somato-sensory pathways in man, EEG clin.Neurophysiol.,
        45:361-375.
Ishikawa, T., McDowall, D. G., 1981, Electrical activity of the
        cerebral cortex during induced hypotension with sodium nitro-
        prusside and trimetaphan in the cat, Br.J. Anaesth.,
        53:605-610.
Jones, T. H., Chiappa, K. H., Young, R. R., Ojemann, R. G., and
        Crowell, R. M., 1979, EEG monitoring for induced hypotension
        for surgery of intracranial aneurysms, Stroke, 10:292-294.
Malnone, M., Prior, P., Scholtz, C. L., 1981, Brain damage after
        cardiopulmonary by-pass: correlations between neurophysio-
        logical and neuropathological findings, J.Neurol.Neurosurg.
        Psychiat., 44:924-931.
Maynard, D., Prior, P. F., and Scott. D. F. 1969. Device for cont-
        inuous monitoring of cerebral activity in resuscitated
        patients, Br.med.J., 4:545-546.
Morris, P. J., Heuser, D., and McDowall, 1982, Controlled hypotension
        in neuroanaesthesia, This volume.
Patel, H., 1981, Experience with the cerebral function monitor during
        deliberate hypotension, Br.J. Anaesth., 53:639-645.
Prior, P., 1979, in: "Monitoring Cerebral Function," P. Prior, ed.,
        Elsevier/North Holland, Amsterdam.
Symon, L., Hargadine, J., Zawirski, M., and Branston, N., 1979,
        Central conduction time as an index of ischaemia in subarach-
        noid haemorrhage, J.Neurol.Sci., 44:94-103.

CRITICAL COMPARISON OF MONITORING EEG, CEREBRAL FUNCTION (CFM),
COMPRESSED SPECTRAL ARRAY (CSA) AND EVOKED RESPONSE UNDER
CONDITIONS OF REDUCED CEREBRAL PERFUSION

P. F. Prior

St. Bartholomew's Hospital
London, EC1A 7BE

This section concerns electrical activity during systemic hypotension in neuro-anaesthesia. My task is to compare the various
methods for recording such activity to warn of inadequate perfusion.
Firstly we must examine the scientific basis for using the brain's
electrical activity as a monitor of cerebral ischaemia. We must
define the characteristics of the relevant electrical changes and
then consider what general methods of displaying them best suit
different clinical or research purposes. There are two broad groups
of monitoring methods: firstly those based on the spontaneous EEG
and secondly those utilizing cerebral potentials evoked by specific
external stimuli. Both spontaneous and evoked activites are only
maintained in their normal form when there is adequate oxidative
neuronal metabolism.

RATIONALE FOR NEUROPHYSIOLOGICAL MONITORING

The EEG gives a direct and non-invasive measure of aspects of
neuronal function that relate closely to level consciousness,
cerebral blood flow (CBF) and metabolism. It has been described as
a "final common denominator" of cerebral perfusion and oxygenation
which continuously reflects changes in cortical function within
seconds. This contrasts with measures such as systemic arterial
pressure, arterial blood gases or end-expired PCO_2 whose relation-
ships to cerebral function are less direct, less immediate and less
all-encompassing. This is illustrated by the value of having a
direct monitor for cortical ischaemic changes during hypotensive
anaesthesia for intracranial aneurysm surgery. The patient may be at
risk because of previous hypertension, unsuspected vertebro-basilar
arterial disease or failure of auto-regulation of CBF following

117

subarachnoid hemorrhage. Systemic arterial pressure surveillance
alone will not indicate when any or all of these adversely affecting
CBF, whereas an EEG monitor will indicate the point when controlled
hypotension begins to depress neuronal function.

Electrical Activity During Cerebral Ischaemia

The classical EEG alteration during an ischaemic episode is
development of abnormality progressing to electrical silence. In a
normal waking EEG during syncope, for example, the alpha and fast
rhythms are replaced by slow waves; then all activity disappears
during unconsciousness. As the circulation recovers large amplitude
slow waves reappear first and then higher frequency, lower amplitude
activity regains its dominance. During anaesthesia a more common
sign of impending ischaemia is development of "burst suppression"
pattern in the EEG (Meldrum and Brierley, 1969). Bursts of waves
(of any frequency) are separated by increasing periods of electrical
silence. The two patterns, EEG slowing and burst suppression activity, may co-exist during onset of perfusion. Both herald electrical silence, the rate of EEG decline depending on the speed and
severity of the perfusion failure. Electrical silence occurs when a
critical threshold for a particular patient has been reached. The
spontaneous EEG becomes silent first and the evoked potentials
slightly later. The sequence of changes affecting the cortical
evoked potentials is mainly one of reduction amplitude and then loss
of the components arising in the cerebral cortex. There is usually
retention of the more robust potentials arising peripherally in the
stimulated nerve which may be recorded in a "far field" manner from
scalp electrodes.

Thresholds for Ischaemic Damage

Shapiro (1978) has summarized these thresholds schematically,
from data in the literature, in terms of oxygenation and perfusion.
He indicates that EEG and evoked potentials begin to alter when PaO_2
is about 40 mmHg, PvO_2 about 28-25 mmHg, CBF 25-20 ml/100g/min and
cerebral perfusion pressure (CPP) below 50 mmHg. The EEG is
abolished when PaO_2 is between 30-25 mmHg, PvO_2 19-17 mmHg, CBF 19-15
ml/100g/min and CPP 40-25 mmHg (i.e. well below the lower limit for
autoregulation of CBF). The evoked potentials survive slightly
longer until CBF has fallen to below 15 ml/100g/min and CPP below
20 mmHg. Of course such figures have to be considered as general
guidelines and the effect of underlined combinations of oxygenation and perfusion deficits borne in mind. Thus pure hypoxic hypoxia to these
levels may not impair cerebral electrical activity directly but only
when it leads to cardio-respiratory embarrassment and associated
reduction in CPP (Brierley et al., 1978). Similarly the supposed
threshold values based on studies in healthy young laboratory animals

or in focal ischaemia, such as during carotid occlusion in man, may need modification before being applied to controlled hypotension in patients undergoing neuroanaesthesia.

In middle cerebral artery occlusion models in primates, Astrup et al. (1977) have shown that there is, in effect, a double threshold for cerebral ischaemia. The first, at CBF of about 15 ml/100g/min is that of electrical failure: this is reversible. The second, when CBF has fallen further, is when potassium leaves neurones and they are irreversibly damaged by ischaemia. Morawetz et al. (1978, 1979) have amplified these threshold concepts indicating that there is a factor of time as well as absolute flow level. Their studies in middle cerebral occlusion in monkeys have shown that electrical silence at steady flows about 12ml/100g/min had to be sustained for two hours before neuronal damage occured. With shorter periods the animals recovered without clinical or neuropathological evidence of infarction.

In global brain ischaemia in the Rhesus monkey due to profound hypotension induced primarily by trimetaphan, Brierley et al. (1969) showed that both EEG and evoked potential silence occured when CPP fell below 25 mmHg. However ischaemic brain damage only occurred if electrical silence was sustained for at least 15 minutes. Furthermore even in animals with quite large infarcts there was, after a delay, recovery of both the spontaneous and evoked activity.

In man cerebral electrical activity reflects factors about ischaemic thresholds demonstrated experimentally. In 25 patients undergoing cardiac surgery at St. Bartholomew's Hospital we observed the behavior of cerebral electrical activity at the onset of bypass. In the 19 in which EEG activity declined (momentarily and never to silence) arterial pressure was significantly lower than in the remainder. Where necessary prompt action was taken to increase pressure and none had neurological complications. Furthermore the EEG decline occurred at higher arterial pressures in older subjects and, as Fitch et al., (1975) have noted experimentally, in those with preoperative hypertension.

These groups of experimental and clinical observations illustrate the rationale for clinical monitoring during controlled hypotension. When cerebral perfusion is insufficient for the requirements of an individual subject there is a warning period of electrical decline and then silence. During this time effective action can be taken to prevent permanent ischaemic damage. Moreover the identification of such cerebral insults from inadequate cerebral perfusion may only be possible by use of neurophysiological monitoring at the time they occur. Post-operatively neurological, psychological, EEG and evoked potential examinations can be entirely normal in the presence of the smaller infarcts (Blagbrough et al., 1973; Brierley et al., 1980).

Distribution Pattern of Ischaemic Brain Damage

Following profound systemic hypotension, ischaemic damage primarily affects the cerebral cortex and may also involve the basal
ganglia. Hypotensive cortical damage has a very specific distribution because of patterns of vulnerability due to vascular factors
(Zulch and Behrend, 1961). The boundary zones between the territories of the main cerebral arteries are the areas at risk: there is a
triple boundary zone in the parietal region at the junction of
posterior, middle and anterior artery territories. This is the site
of the minimal infarct and ischaemic damage is always maximal there.
With more severe infarcts cortical damage spreads forwards parasagit-
tally along the anterior-middle and, to a lesser extent, laterally
along the middle-posterior cerebral artery boundary zones. It
generally spares the frontal poles and temporal lobes. This distribution of brain damage in the arterial boundary zones is quite commonly encountered clinically due to reduced systemic or raised intracranial pressure or both (Brierley and Miller, 1966; Adams et al.,
1966; Graham, 1977). The pattern of ischaemic damage will also be
affected by underlying local occlusive vascular disease in the neck
or intracranially (Yates and Hutchinson, 1961). In patients undergoing hypotensive anaesthesia neither occlusive vascular disease nor
the effects of age or previous arterial hypertension on the lower
limit for autoregulation may be predictable preoperatively. This is
a strong argument for routine EEG monitoring, because of the difficulty of predicting the precise effect on cerebral perfusion of
factors such as posture and peripheral pooling in patients who may
have a reduced capacity for autoregulation of CBF.

Relationship Between Depression of Electrical Activity and Severity
of Ischaemic Damage

Neuropathological studies of arterial boundary zone infarcts
demonstrate the relationship between depression of electrical activity and severity of subsequent ischaemic damage. Malone et al.,
(1981) reported 20 patients dying up to 3 years after cardiac surgery
with bypass who had been examined neuropathologically. Nine had, and
11 had not, clinical evidence of brain damage and all had had operative monitoring of cerebral electrical activity. The presence and
extent of boundary zone infarction found in all 9 with neurological
deficit was related to severity of operative EEG depression during
periods of presumed hypoperfusion, due to severe hemorrhage, major
cardiac arrhythmias or profound hypotension. Infarcts only occured
when major EEG depression had exceeded 7 min followed by slow or
partial recovery. The severity of EEG depression was also related to
the degree of clinical deficit as reported earlier in a larger group
of patients from the same unit (Schwartz et al., 1973). Short
periods (less than 7 minutes) of electrical depression with rapid
recovery were followed by a normal neurological state and when the

patient subsequentyly died from cardiac disease, a brain without
evidence of infarction.

Similar findings are reported in animal models of arterial
boundary zone infarcts for example due to profound arterial hypotension (Brierley et al., 1969). More recently Brierley et al.
(1980) reduced cerebral hemisphere perfusion in lightly anaes-
thetised, spontaneously breathing baboons by temporary, sequential
bilateral common carotid artery occlusion. Moderate hypoxia (PaO_2
about mmHg) had abolished autoregulation. The EEG were scored
visually using a simple 6-point scale representing the change from
continuous EEG (1) through increasing burst suppression activity
(2-5) to electrical silence (6) (Prior et al., 1979). The minute-
by-minute sequential scores below the baseline anaesthetic level
were summed during ischaemia and the immediate recovery period.
The higher the score the more severe the EEG depression. When EEG
silence exceeded 8 min, brain damage was always found in the arterial
boundary zones. There was a close correlation between the EEG
scores and quantified histological assessment of the extent and
severity of the brain damage. In a sub-group of 4 animals (Brierley
and Prior, unpublished data) trimetaphan reduced the substantial
reflex hypertension induced by the bilateral common carotid occlusion. External doppler (Dr. M. Lunt, St. Bartholomew's Hospital;
Hauge et al., 1980) demonstrated loss of vertebral artery flow during
the time that trimetaphan-induced hypotension led to prolonged EEG
silence. Cerebral damage was very severe in these 4 animals, in 2
amounting to brain death indicating the considerable risk of induced
hypotension in the presence of vascular occlusion.

WHAT TYPE OF CEREBRAL MONITORING

Having discussed the general relevance of the techniques as
cerebral monitors the practical methods must now be considered.

Choice Between Evoked Potentials and EEG

Several anatomical and pathological factors are pertinent when
considering the optimal method for monitoring during neurosurgical
procedures. The risk of focal or of global ischaemia or some combination of the two defines not only sites for recording electrodes
but whether evoked potentials or spontaneous EEG are appropriate.

Because induced hypotension per se leads to global reduction
in CBF especially in the arterial boundary zone regions, adequacy of
cerebral perfusion is best monitored by EEG recording from electrodes placed over these areas. If temporary arterial occlusion is
part of the neurosurgical procedure either local EEG recording in the
territory of the artery involved or evoked potentials may also be
necessary.

When a middle cerebral artery is occluded, as in the baboons
studied by Symon et al. (1976), the infarct is usually restricted to
deep structures around the internal capsule and the cortex is normal.
However the somato-sensory potentials evoked by electrical stimulation of a peripheral nerve traverse the relevant area; their cortical appearance will be affected by any intervening lesion inter-
rupting their pathway. Thus evoked potential recordings may be expected on anatomical grounds to give the best monitor for neurosurgical procedures involving specific neural pathways. They may
also prove to be more reliable than EEG during carotid artery
surgery.

Evoked Potentials

     Cerebral evoked potentials are very small indeed and are virtu-
ally undetectable by eye amongst the spontaneous cortical EEG
rhythms.   For this reason one must record following a large number
(often a few hundred up to a thousand or more) or rapidly presented
stimuli.   If there is no response evoked, superimposed EEG recordings
starting from the stimulu will not show any consistent pattern.   In
contrast an evoked response with a constant time relationship to the
stimulus will build up and stand out clearly.   Modern apparatus
generally averages rather than superimposes these evoked potentials.

     Potentials evoked by peripheral somatosensory stimulation (e.g.
an electrical stimulus to a median nerve) can be recorded at spinal,
brainstem and cortical levels.   Their transit time for upper spine to
contralateral sensory cortex is of the order of 5-6 msec and has been
designated the "central somatosensory conduction time".   It has
proved a useful measure in neurosurgery.   Hume, Shaw and Cant (1979)
demonstrated that it is independent of arm length, temperature or
anaesthetic depth and is increased with post traumatic oedema.   Symon
(this volume) has indicated its relevance as an index of ischaemia in
patients after subarachnoid haemmorhage.

     The main advantage of evoked potentials compared to the EEG is
the ease of obtaining objective measurements.   Furthermore, auto-
mation of the measurement with indication of deviations from normal,
is possible (Billings, 1981).   It must be emphasised that there are
considerable problems in using evoked potentials as clinical monitors
during neurosurgery.   They have 4 general disadvantages: firstly,
they only represent one very specific localized event, or pathway;
secondly, they give only an intermittent measurment because of the
time necessary for accumulating the average; thirdly, they are very
demanding technically because of the very small brief potentials
involved and fourthly, the cortical potentials (but not the brainstem
or central conduction ones) are affected considerably by anaesthesia.
The use of evoked potentials as monitors for detection of ischaemia
is presently mainly confined to research studies, although some

neurosurgical units find them valuable for other purposes, such as
visual evoked potentials during the dissection of chiasmal lesions,
auditory brainstem potentials during posterior fossa procedures or
somato-sensory potentials during spinal surgery.

Spontaneous EEG

For all its complexity and the voluminous nature of traditional
paper tracings, the EEG has the unique attribute of giving continuous
information about brain function which can be obtained noninvasively.
It is quite amenable to simple data reduction and quantification by
rating scales of the type described earlier. Such rating is more
appropriate in a research setting where it can usually be performed
retrospectively, either visually or by computer analysis of tape-
recorded data. For clinical monitoring the situation is different
and one must look to some sort of immediate and automatic processing
to reject artefacts and highlight relevant features in the EEG, if
possible putting them into digital or an easily measurable form.

Three main groups of technique have emerged, each with one
commercial version available. Traditional analysis methods include
those considering EEG frequency and those considering EEG amplitude.
Recently a number of methods have appeared which combine the advantages of both.

Frequency can be measured in various ways. Analogue filters can
be tuned to various bands, fast Fourier transforms disclose the
frequency spectra or repeated baseline crossing counts can give
duration (i.e. period) of each wave allowing calculation of frequency
content. The Fourier transform method is described as a frequency
domain and the period analysis as a time domain. Frequency methods
all have the basic disadvantage, as with evoked potentials, that they
require a finite time segment of EEG for analysis. This means sum-
marizing the events in epochs ranging, say, from 4 to 60 seconds.
Brief events, for example short silent periods in early burst suppression, are lost. The methods usually display sequential summaries
of frequency measurements which resemble contour maps. These displays may further mask brief events because of superimposition.

The Fourier methods are exemplified by the compressed spectral
array (CSA) of Bickford et al. (1973) which is also the basis of the
commercially available Berg Fourier Analyzer. Two channels (one for
each hemisphere) can be processed simultaneously. The density modulated spectral array (DSA) of Fleming and Smith (1979) is a variation
of this method whereby graded scale dots replace the lines, with the
reported advantage of less obscuration of later events than in the
linear CSA display. With both these methods it is easy to see when
a major event occurs such as a marked frequency alteration or loss
of virtually all EEG activity. The early frequency changes with

perfusion failure may be more subtle and difficult for the non-elec-
troencephalographer to see and interpret on CSA or DSA displays.
Frequency information has been an obsession of electroencephalo-
graphers since the early 1930s and indeed it has much to say about
subtle changes in anaesthetic depth. But it is unnecessarily complex
and at times even confusing for ischaemia monitoring. Furthermore
there is no evidence at present that infarction occurs where there
has been frequency change alone. Myers et al. (1977) have illustrated a comparison between CSA and integrated amplitude displays
during a period of reduced cerebral perfusion. The simple amplitude
measure appears to provide a more straightforward and easily measurable warning of ischaemic depression of EEG. Integrated amplitude
(pioneered by Drohocki, 1938) falls into the time domain analysis and
permits a continuous display of cerebral event. This is very important in clinical monitoring.

     The cerebral function monitor (CFM) of Maynard et al. (1969),
which is also available commercially, is a simpler and cheaper (by a
factor of 5 or 6) apparatus than the CSA. It gives a continuous
display of EEG amplitude variations from minimum to maximum. The
compressed write out of the CFM is thus a band rather like that of
arterial blood pressure, in contrast to integrated amplitude which
gives a linear display. The degree of amplitude variation is very
informative clinically and is particularly suited to displaying burst
suppression activity which gives a low level band ranging from zero
microvolts during total suppressions to peaks with amplitude proportional to that of the bursts of activity. The processing of the EEG
signal includes some filtering and artefact rejection to reduce the
various forms of interference which are a common problem in the
operating theater and one often, surprisingly poorly overcome with
other systems. In the CFM there is also a continuous write out of
the integrity of the electrode connections and circuitry.

     Clinically it is helpful to monitor cerebral activity on the
same chart as systemic factors such as arterial pressure and heart
rate. During induced hypotension such polygraphic monitoring (Figure
1) will indicate when a critical arterial pressure for a particular
patient is reached and the CFM amplitude starts to fall as CBF becomes pressure dependent. Ishikawa and McDowall (1981) have shown in
the cat, a linear relationship between mean CFM level and mean arterial pressure when the latter is below the lower limit for autoregulation: the CFM fall parallels falling CBF. A similar relationship
exists in man (Patel, 1981)

     Recording from scalp electrodes is technically satisfactory
during neurosurgical intervention (Figure 1). It is also possible
to record separately from special electrocorticography electrodes
direct on the brain in the territory of the vessel being operated
upon but out of the surgical field. This allows a convenient division of responsibility between the neurosurgeon with his clamp

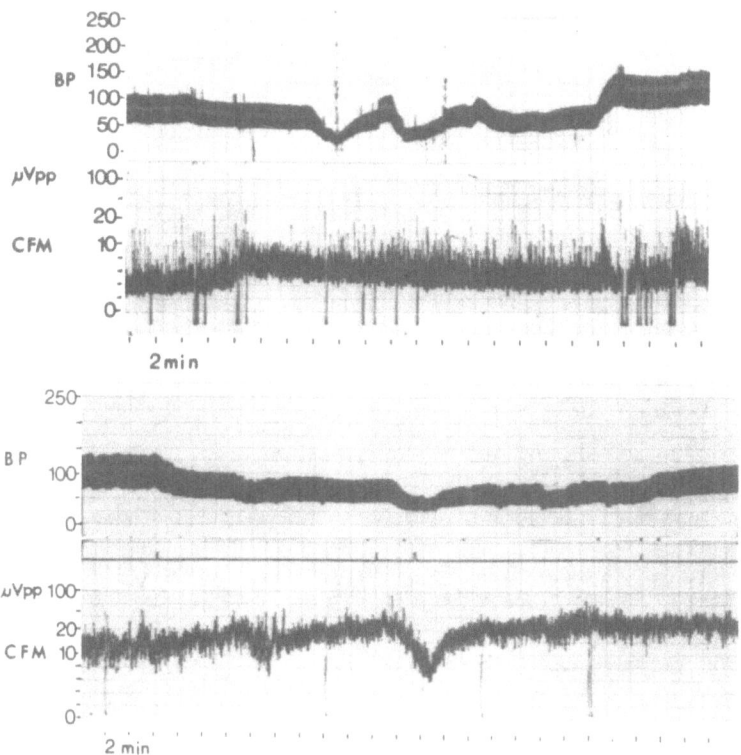

Fig. 1. Polygraphic recordings of arterial blood pressure (BP) and
CFM in two patients during clipping of intracranial aneurysms. In the upper recording cerebral activity is stable
during the period of most profound (nitroprusside-induced)
hypotension whilst the aneurysm is prepared for clipping.
In contrast in the lower recording, lesser falls in arterial
pressure are mirrored by dips in the CFM trace due to impaired autoregulation following subarachnoid hemorrhage.
Immediate reduction in nitroprusside allows pressure to rise
and the CFM recovers. (Recordings of D. Hardy and P. O'Shea
modified from Prior, 1979).

producing local ischaemia and the anaesthetist with his controlled
hypotension producing global ischaemia. Two separate chart recorders
are necessary or some system for multiplexing or alternating the two
recordings.

It can be argued that a combination of EEG amplitude and frequency features will give the optimal information for monitoring,
providing the display is sufficiently straightforward. One method is
illustrated (Figures 2 and 3) with data recorded during cardiac
surgery by Etherington (1981).

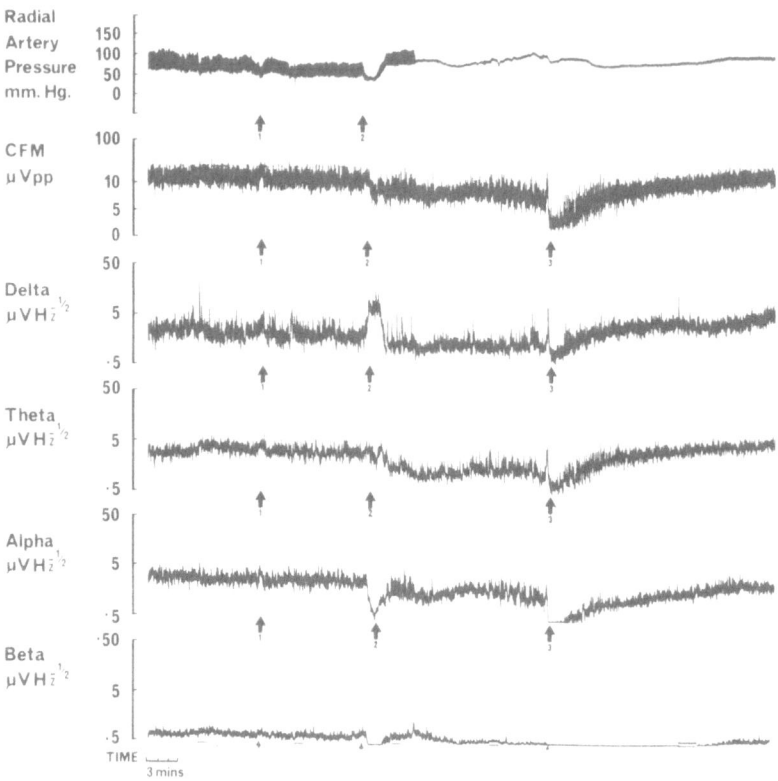

Fig. 2. Arterial pressure and CFM are displayed with root mean
         square (r.m.s.) power spectral densities in the orthodox
         frequency bands obtained by selective filtering of the
         raw EEG output from the CFM. Transient falls in arterial
         pressure (arrows 1 and 2) occur before and at the start
         of cardiopulmonary bypass. This is followed by cooling to
         30°C and (arrow 3) a bolus injection of Althesin 2 ml.

     Two other forms of combined frequency and amplitude monitor
have been proposed. These are the period-amplitude display of Davis
and Klein (1977) and a development of the CFM by Maynard (1977). The
latter is a modified, microprocessor-controlled CFM, the CFAM,
(Figure 4) which is shortly becoming available commercially at quite
modest cost. It has several new features of particular interest.
Firstly, it analyses the voltage trace of the standard CFM to give
backwards weighted average values for the maximum, mean and minimum
amplitudes, whilst retaining individual peaks and troughs. The scale
is fully logarithmic and the frequency range has been increased to
2-27 Hz. Secondly, frequency analysis by a multiple baseline crossing and integrating procedure (a type of period analysis) has been
used. The third feature, not illustrated, is a facility to interrupt
recording and average and display 2-channel evoked potentials with

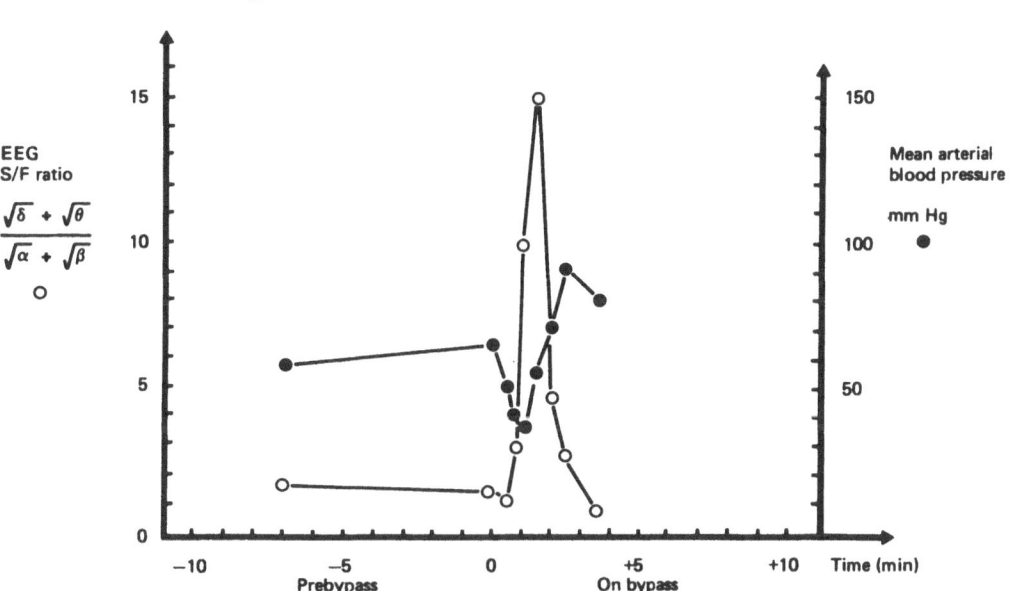

Fig. 3. Data from Figure 2 has been converted into the ratio
between slow and fast r.m.s. power spectral densities
$(\frac{delta + theta}{alpha + beta})$ and plotted against arterial pressures.
Such ratios can be computed and displayed on line with
relatively cheap methods and may well provide a valuable
supplement to other displays.

appropriate scaling for both cortical and brainstem events on the
same chart. The same microprocessor permits other computations such
as trend analysis and generates digital data. This flexibility makes
the CFAM likely to be a very attractive proposition as a multi-
purpose clinical monitor.

Critical Comparison Between EEG Monitoring Methods

In order to choose whether any one type of EEG monitoring method
is superior for a particular purpose it is necessary to compare
the performance of those available with the same (usually tape recorded) data. Such comparisons generally require a considerable
amount of data for statistical validity. Discussion in the anaesthetic literature on the relative merits or de-merits of various
monitors in the last few years has been intemperate, partisan and
anecdotal. Controversy has related to methods of processing and
displaying the EEG as a monitor, that is arguments between frequency
and amplitude analyses of the two and between types of frequency
analysis method and of display (e.g. Levy et al., 1980).

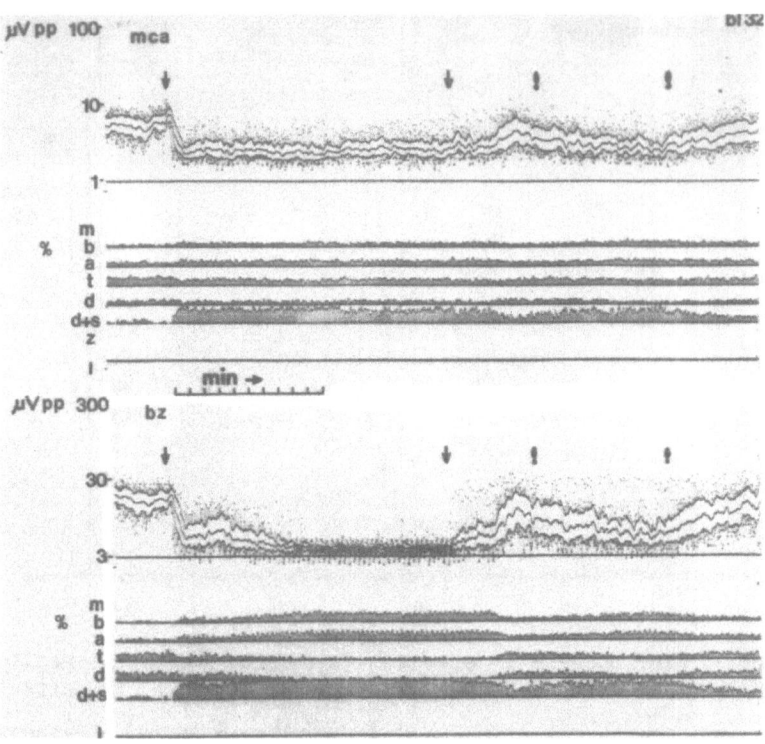

Fig. 4.   CFAM recording of ischaemic episode in a baboon to compare
          cortical electrodes in central territory of the middle
          cerebral artery (mca) and at the boundary zone (bz) between
          middle and anterior cerebral arteries. Analyzed amplitude
          traces (see text) and scalp muscle potentials (M) the pro-
          portions of activities in each of the EEG frequency bands
          (b = beta, a = alpha, t = theta, d = delta), delta at less
          than 1 Hz together with suppressions (d+s), z = electrode
          impedance and 1 = mains interference. Bilateral cerebral
          hemisphere ischaemia produced during hypoxia (PaO$_2$ 23-24
          mmHg PaCO$_2$ 34 mmHg) in lightly anaesthetized spontaneously
          breathing animal by 19 minutes bilateral common carotid
          artery occlusion (between arrows). The more severe EEG
          change occurs at the bz where small parietal infarcts were
          subsequently demonstrated. The bz increase in faster com-
          ponents during ischaemia shows how misleading a mean fre-
          quency measure would be. Between the two marks on the right
          is the effect of increasing Althesin infusion from 0.63 to
          0.93 ml/kg/hr.

     There has been more objective critical comparison of methods on
a statistical basis in the neurophysiological literature to which one
should refer for methodological details. Surveys of the basic

methods of analysis will be found in the Handbook of Electroencephalography and Clinical Neurophysiology (1972, 1973), Rémond (1977)
and Cooper et al. (1980). Statistical comparisons of different
methods which have set methodological standards include those of
Matousek et al. (1978) and Matthis et al. (1981). Data during cardiopulmonary bypass (Pronk et al., 1980) and during focal ischaemic
episodes (Tolonen and Sulg, 1981) have been the subject of similar
careful analyses. The concensus view is that frequency methods are
more sensitive to subtle EEG change than amplitude ones but this
relative advantage is offset by their greater complexity and sensitivity to artefact and to fluctuating levels of consciousness.
However testing of the amplitude methods was somewhat limited in most
of these studies. Power spectral and frequency ratio methods had
slight theoretical advantages over the period analysis or filtering
methods, but generally speaking the differences were not gross.

None of the studies in either anaesthetic or EEG literature has
yet an adequate comparison between available monitoring methods for
detection of ischaemia due to controlled hypotension in neuroanaesthesia. It is clear that the complex frequency methods have
more to offer for monitoring anaesthetic depth, whilst the simpler
amplitude methods provide the most clear cut warning of cerebral
ischaemia. The combined methods, such as period-amplitude display or
the CFAM, are likely to provide the most versatile clinical tools.
The addition or substitution of evoked potential measures such as
central somatosensory conduction time may be helpful for certain
neurosurgical procedures. However, the most important decision is to
incorporate some form of functional brain monitoring technique as a
warning of when cerebral perfusion is reduced to a critical threshold
for an individual patient so that arterial pressure can be increased
before ischaemic damage occurs. The arguments between different
types of cerebral monitor are minor compared with those in favor of
the use of such monitoring as a routine during controlled hypotension
in neuroanaesthesia.

REFERENCES

Adams, J. H., Brierley, J. B., Connor, R. C. R., and Treip, C. S.,
    1966, The effects of systemic hypotension upon the human
    brain, Brain, 89:235.
Astrup, J., Symon, L., Branston, N. M., and Lassen, N. A., 1977,
    Cortical evoked potential and extracellular K^+ and H^+ at
    critical levels of brain ischaemia, Stroke, 8:51.
Bickford, R. G., Brimm, J., Berger, L., and Aung, M., 1973, Appli-
    cation of compressed spectral array in clinical EEG, in:
    "Automation of Clinical Electroencephalography," P. Kellaway
    and I. Petersen, eds., Raven Press, New York, 55.
Billings, R. J., 1981, Automatic detection, measurement and documen-
    tation of the visual evoked potential using a commercial

microprocessor-equipped averager, Electroenceph.Clin.
     Neurophysiol., 52:214.
Blagbrough, A. E., Brierley, J. B., and Nicholson, A. N., 1973,
     Behavioural and neurological disturbances associated with
     hypoxic brain damage, J.Neurol.Sci., 18:475.
Brierley, J. B., and Miller, A. A., 1966, Fatal brain damage after
     dental anaesthesia. Its nature, aetiology and prevention,
     Lancet, ii:869.
Brierley, J. B., Brown, A. W., Excell, B. J., and Meldrum, B. S.,
     1969, Brain damage in the Rhesus monkey resulting from pro-
     found arterial hypotension. Its nature, distribution and
     general physiological correlates, Brain Res., 13:68.
Brierley, J. B., Prior, P. F., Calverley, J., and Brown, A. W., 1978,
     Profound hypoxia in Papio anubis and Macaca mulatta - physio-
     logical and neuropathological effects, J.Neurol.Sci., 37:1.
Brierley, J. B., Prior, P. F., Calverley, J., Jackson, S. J., and
     Brown, A. W., 1980, Pathogenesis of ischaemic neuronal damage
     along the cerebral arterial boundary zones in Papio anubis,
     Brain, 103:929.
Cooper, R., Osselton, J. W., and Shaw, J. C., 1980, "EEG Technology,"
     3rd edition, Butterworths, London.
Davis, D. A., and Klein, F. F., 1977, A clinically practical method
     of EEG analysis and its performance under common states of
     anesthesia, Abstract, Annual Meeting of American Society of
     Anesthesiologists.
Drohocki, Z., 1938, L'electrospectrographie du cerveau, C.R. Soc.
     Biol., 129:889.
Etherington, N. J., 1981, Continuous assessment of brain function:
     the design and evaluation of an electroencephalographic fre-
     quency band monitor. M.Sc.Thesis, University of London.
Fleming, R. A., and Smith, N. T., 1979, An inexpensive device for
     analysing and monitoring the electroencephalogram,
     Anesthesiology, 50:456.
Fitch, W., Jones, J. V., Graham, D. I., MacKenzie, E. T., Harper, A.
     M., 1978, Effects of hypotension induced by halothane, on the
     cerebral circulation in baboons with experimental renovascular
     hypotension, Br.J.Anaesth., 50:119.
Graham, D. I., 1977, Pathology of hypoxic damage in man, in: "Hypoxia
     and Ischaemia," B. C. Morson, ed., J.Clin.Path. 30 supplement
     (Royal College of Pathologists), 11:170.
Handbook of Electroencephalography and Clinical Neurophysiology,
     1972, 1973, A. Rémond, ed., vols 4B and 5A, Elsevier, North
     Holland, Amsterdam.
Hange, A., Thoresen, M., and Walløe, L., 1980, Changes in cerebral
     blood flow during hyperventilation and CO_2 breathing measured
     transcutaneously in humans by a bidirectional, pulsed, ultra-
     sound doppler blood velocity meter, Acta Physiol.Scand.,
     110:167.
Hume, A. L., Cant, B. R., and Shaw, N. A., 1979, Central somatosen-
     sory conduction time in comatose patients, Ann.Neurol., 5:379.

Ishikawa, T. and McDowall, D. G., 1981, Electrical activity of the
     cerebral cortex during induced hypotension with sodium nitro-
     prusside and trimetaphan in the cat, Br.J.Anaesth., 53:605.
Levy, W. J., Shapiro, H. M., Maruchak, G., and Meathe, E., 1980,
     Automated EEG processing for intraoperative monitoring,
     Anesthesiology, 53:223.
Malone, M., Prior, P., and Scholtz, C. L., 1981, Brain damage after
     cardiopulmonary by-pass: correlations between neurophysio-
     logical and neuropathological findings, J.Neurol., Neurosurg.,
     Psychiat., 44:924.
Matoušek, M., Arridsson, A., and Friberg, S., 1978, Implementation of
     analytical methods in daily clinical EEG, in: "Contemporary
     Clinical Neurophysiology," W. A. Cobb and H. van Duijn,
     Elsevier, Amsterdam, 199.
Matthis, P., Scheffner, D., and Benninger, C., 1981, Spectral
     analysis of the EEG; comparison of various spectral para-
     meters, Electroenceph.clin.Neurophysiol., 52:218.
Maynard, D. E., 1977, The cerebral function analyser monitor (CFAM),
     Electroenceph.clin.Neurophysiol., 43:479.
Maynard, D., Prior, P. F., and Scott, D. F., 1969, A device for
     continuous monitoring of cerebral activity in resuscitated
     patients, Br.Med.J., 4:545.
Meldrum, B. S., and Brierley, J. B., 1969, Brain damage in the Rhesus
     monkey resulting from profound arterial hypotension. II,
     changes in the spontaneous and evoked electrical activity of
     the neocortex, Brain Res., 13:101.
Morawetz, R. B., Crowell, R. H., de Girolami, U., Marcoux, F. W.,
     Jones, T. H., and Halsey, J. H., 1979, Regional cerebral blood
     flow thresholds during cerebral ischaemia, Fed.Proc., 38:2493.
Morawetz, R. B., de Girolami, U., Ojemann, R. G., Marcoux, F. W., and
     Crowell, R. M., 1978, Cerebral blood flow determined by hy-
     drogen clearance during middle cerebral artery occlusion in
     unanesthetised monkeys, Stroke, 9:331.
Myers, R. R., Stockard, J. J., and Saidman, L. J., 1977, Monitoring
     of cerebral perfusion during anesthesia by time-compressed
     Fourier analysis of the electroencephalogram, Stroke, 8:331.
Patel, H., 1981, Experience with the cerebral function monitor during
     deliberate hypotension, Br.J.Anaesth., 53:639.
Prior, P. F., 1979, "Monitoring Cerebral Function," Elsevier/North
     Holland, Amsterdam.
Prior, P. F., Maynard, D. E., and Brierley, J. B., 1978, EEG monitor-
     ing for the control of anaesthesia produced by the infusion of
     althesin in primates, Br.J.Anaesth., 50:993.
Pronk, R. A. F., Doombos, P., Hengeveld, S. J., Cornelissen, R. C.
     M., Ackerstaff, R. G. A., Simons, A. J. R., and Lopes da
     Silva, F. H., 1980, Automatic recognition of abnormal EEG
     patterns during open heart surgery, Progress Report 7, Inst.
     Med.Phys., Utrecht, 61.
Rémond, A., ed., 1977, "EEG Informatics," Elsevier, Amsterdam.
Shapiro, H. M., 1978, Monitoring in neurosurgical anesthesia, in:

"Monitoring in Anesthesia," L. J. Saidman and N. T. Smith,
    eds., Wiley, New York, 171.
Schwartz, M. S., Colvin, M. P., Prior, P. F., Strunin, L., Simpson,
    B. R., and Weaver, E. J. M., 1973, The cerebral function
    monitor; its value in predicting the neurological outcome in
    patients undergoing cardiopulmonary by-pass, Anaesthesia,
    28:611.
Symon, L., Dorsch, W. W. C., Crockard, H. A., Branston, N. M., and
    Brierley, J. B., 1976, Clinical features, local CBP and vas-
    cular reactivity in a chronic (3-year) stroke in baboons, in:
    "Blood Flow and Metabolism in the Brain," A. M. Harper, W. B.
    Jennett, J. D. Miller, and J. O. Rowan, eds., Churchill
    Livingstone, Edinburgh.
Tolonen, H., Sulg, I. A., 1981, Comparison of quantitative EEG para-
    meters from four different analysis techniques in evaluation
    of relationships between EEG and CBF in brain infarction,
    Electroenceph.clin.Neurophysiol., 51:177.
Yates, P. O., and Hutchinson, E. C., 1961, Cerebral infarction: the
    role of stenosis of the extracranial cerebral arteries,
    MRC Special Report Series, No.300, HMSO, London.
Zülch, K. J. and Behrend, R. C. H., 1961, The pathogenesis and topo-
    graphy of anoxia and ischaemia of the brain in man, in:
    "Cerebral Anoxia and the Electroencephalogram," H. Gastaut and
    J. S. Meyer, eds., Thomas, Illinois, 144.

THE USE OF SOMATOSENSORY EVOKED

POTENTIALS IN NEUROSURGICAL PRACTICE

L. Symon and A. D. J. Wang

Neurological Surgery
Institute of Neurology
Queen Square, London WC1N 3BG

INTRODUCTION

   Changes in evoked electrical activity of the brain are related
to critical reduction in cerebral blood flow both in man and primates
(Trojaborg and Boysen 1973; Branston et al., 1974). Somatosensory
evoked potentials following median nerve stimulation have been found
useful to monitor cerebral ischaemia (Symon et al., 1979; Hargadine
et al., 1980), following subarachnoid hemorrhage and intracranial
aneurysm surgery.

MATERIALS AND METHODS

   The technique employed has been modified from that of Hume and
Cant (Symon et al., 1979; Hume and Cant 1978). The median nerve at
the wrist is stimulated by bipolar electrodes placed over the median
nerve, with the cathode 3 cm proximal to the anode, and square wave
pulses of a stimulus intensity 2-3 times subjective threshold and
just sufficient to elicit a small thumb twitch, and of 0.15 msecs
duration, delivered at a rate of 3 per second. Recording electrodes
over the C2 spine and over the somatosensory cortex (C3/C4), with a
frontal reference Fpz, have been used. 256 or 512 sweeps were averaged, using a Medelec MS6 or a Digitimer D200 system.

   Central conduction time (CCT), that is the interval between the
N13/14 wave at C2 and the N20 wave at the somatosensory cortex, was
measured from both hemispheres in patients with subarachnoid hemorrhage and radiologically demonstrable aneurysms, who were to undergo
surgical intervention. The first study involved pre and postoperative recordings, and more recently preoperative studies have also been

made. The clinical status was judged by one of us (LS) on the Hunt
and Hess scale. Outcome was defined at two months as either good,
that is patients who had full activity with no or minimal neurological deficit, or poor, patients who either died or were unable to work
from neurological deficit or requiring long term care.

Thirteen patients with subarachnoid hemorrhage, but with no
neurological signs and no radiologically demonstrable aneurysm, were
used as a control group. The mean CCT of this group was not dissimilar from that of normal volunteers (Symon et al., 1979), and was 5.4
± 0.4 msecs. A CCT of more than 6.4 msecs, (mean + 2.5 standard
deviations), was taken as the level of significantly prolonged conduction time. Recordings were taken preoperatively, postoperatively
within one day of surgery, at 48-72 hours, on the fifth postoperative
day and in the second week. Preoperative recording was started when
the patient was under anaesthetic during induction, was followed
throughout the operation and finished with a recording in the recovery room as the patient regained consciousness.

Table 1. CCT of Patients According to Preoperative Status

Hemisphere/preoperative grade	Grade 0+I	Grade II	Grade III	Grade IV
Affected hemisphere	5.8 ± 0.6 (n=6)	5.7 ± 0.5 (n=27)	5.8 ± 0.6 (n=21)	6.3 ± 0.7 (n=14)
Unaffected hemisphere	5.7 ± 9.5 (n=6)	5.7 ± 0.4 (n=26)	5.7 ± 0.4 (n=21)	6.1 ± 0.4 (n=14)

Table 2. CCT of Patients According to Outcome

Outcome	Time interval Hemisphere	Preop	Day 1	48-72 hr	Day 5	2 Week
GOOD	Affected	5.7±9.5 (n=58)	6.0±0.6 (n=44)	6.0±0.5 (n=45)	5.9±0.6 (n=29)	5.8±0.5 (n=36)
	Unaffected	5.7±0.7 (n=52)	5.8±0.5 (n=43)	5.8±0.5 (n=47)	5.7±0.5 (n=32)	5.6±0.5 (n=35)
POOR	Affected	6.3±0.7 (n=14)	6.8±1.9 (n=10)	6.7±2.0 (n=11)	6.5±1.6 (n=11)	6.7±1.3 (n=12)
	Unaffected	5.9±0.4 (n=14)	5.9±0.6 (n=12)	5.8±0.5 (n=13)	6.0±0.5 (n=14)	5.6±1.6 (n=13)

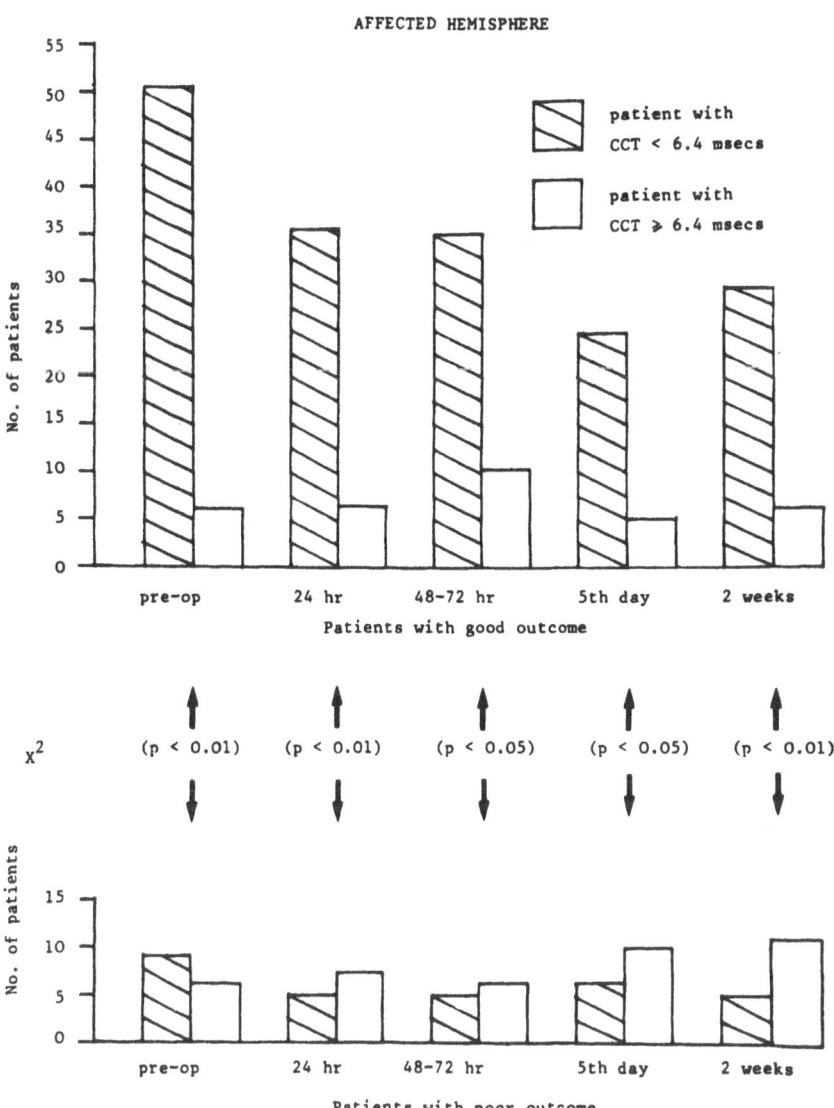

Fig. 1.   Histogram distribution of patients with either normal or
          abnormal CCT (>6.4 msecs) in the subgroup of good and poor
          outcome.   Significant differences showed in each time
          interval.

RESULTS

Pre and Post Operative Recording

Serial CCT measurements were made in 79 patients with subarachnoid hemorrhage from angiographically proven aneurysm, aged 22–68
years, 23 being male and 56 female. The mean CCT values of the
patients according to preoperative clinical status is shown in
Table 1. CCT was recorded from the affected hemisphere, that is the

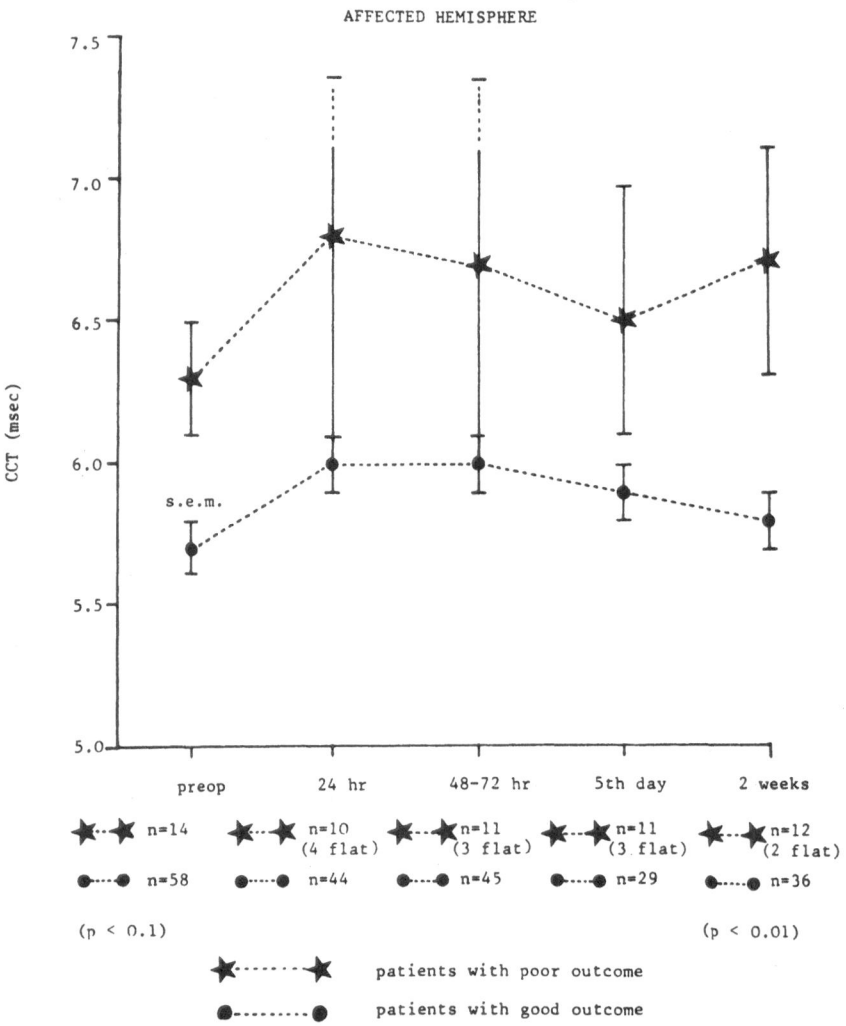

Fig. 2.   Diagram of mean CCT change in each time interval according
          to outcome, the preoperation CCT and CCT in second week
          showed significant differences in two subgroups (p<0.01).

Table 3.   Interhemispheric Difference According to Outcome

Time interval Outcome	Preop	Day 1	48-72 Hr	Day 5	2 Week
GOOD	0.4 ± 0.4 (n=53)	0.4 ± 0.3 (n=42)	0.4 ± 0.3 (n=38)	0.5 ± 0.4 (n=30)	0.4 ± 0.3 (n=29)
POOR	0.5 ± 0.5 (n=14)	0.7 ± 1.4 (n=8)	1.1 ± 1.7 (n=9)	0.7 ± 1.2 (n=11)	0.8 ± 1.1 (n=13)

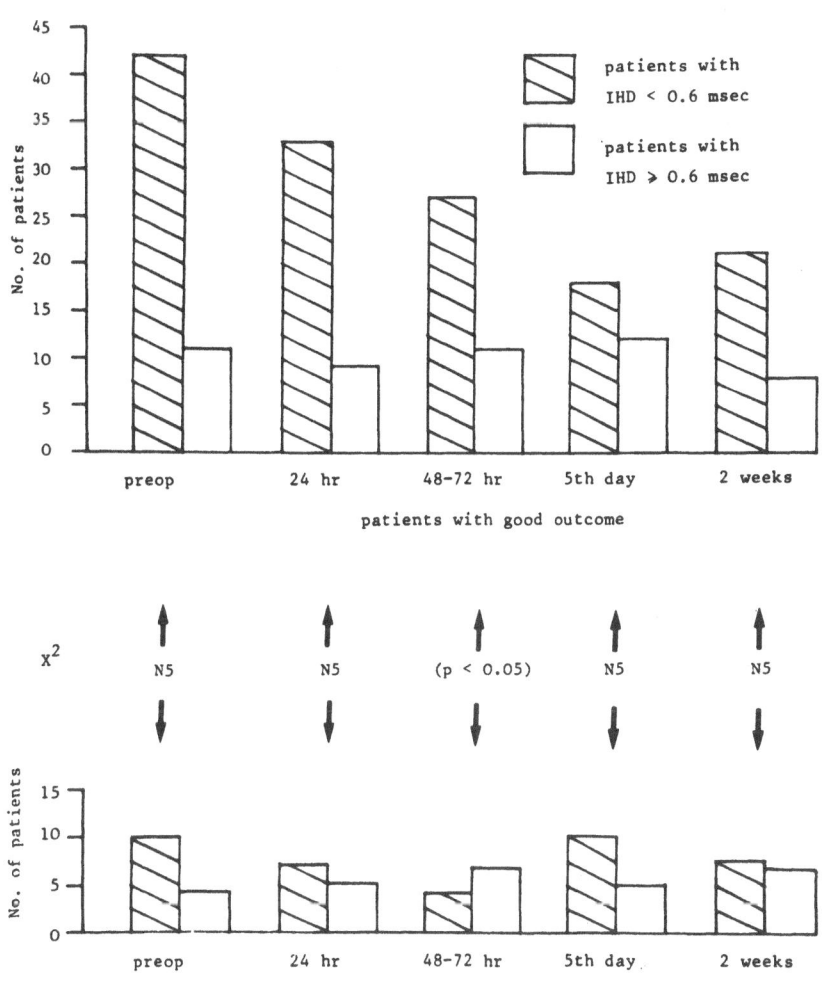

Fig. 3.   Histogram distribution of patients with normal or abnormal
(>0.6 msecs) interhemispheric difference in the subgroup of
good and poor outcome. Note that the 48-72 hour time showed
significant difference.

aneurysm-bearing hemisphere or the hemisphere related to any neurological deficit in midline aneurysm, such as anterior communicating
or basilar, was significantly prolonged in grade 4 patients. The
mean (6.3 ± 0.7 msecs) was statistically different from the control
group (p<0.01, n = 14).

CCT as a Prognostic Indicator

Table 2 shows the CCT of groups with good and poor outcome in
the affected and unaffected hemispheres, and Figure 1 the histogram
distribution of patients with either normal or abnormal CCT in the
subgroups of good and poor outcome. There is statistically significant difference by T test, (p<0.010 between prolonged CCT in the
preoperative period, and outcome; and between prolonged CCT in the
second week and outcome, p<0.01) (Figure 2). The distribution histogram between the two subgroups is significant at all time intervals.
Interhemispheric difference was also measured between the affected

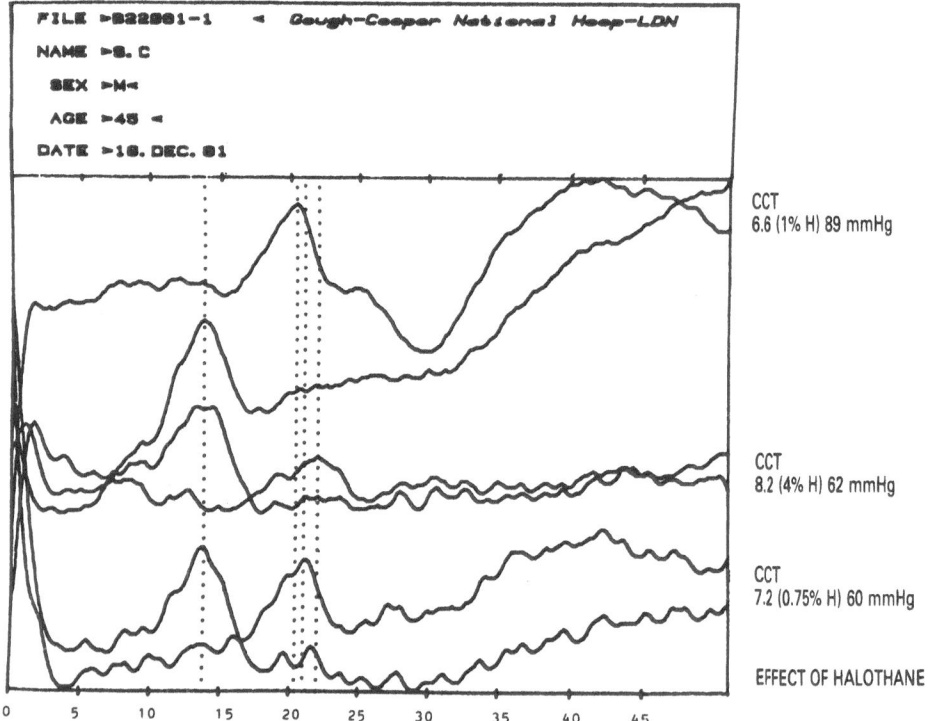

Fig. 4a. CCT change after change of halothane concentration. CCT
          increased up to 8.2 msecs from 6.6 msecs when halothane
          increased from 1% to 4% and returned to 7.2 msec when
          halothane reduced to 0.75%.

and unaffected hemispheres, and Table 3 shows that there is a tendency for poor outcome cases to show an interhemispheric difference
longer than 0.6 msecs. (Mean + two standard deviations of the norm.)
The distribution of prolonged interhemispheric difference is significant at the 48-72 hour time recording (p<0.05) (Figure 3).

Preoperative Recording

Fifteen aneurysm cases have been recorded throughout operation,
the position of the indifferent and recording electrodes being such
that they can be maintained in satisfactory position away from the
small fronto-temporal craniotomy around the outer end of the sphen-
oidal wing routinely used in this department. Several interesting
facts have emerged from preoperative recording. The introduction of
Halothane into the anaesthetic circuit produced significant prolongation of CCT from a preoperative mean of 6.0 ± 0.6 msecs to 6.8 ± 0.6
msecs (p<0.05)   (Figure 4a and b). The actual turning of the bone

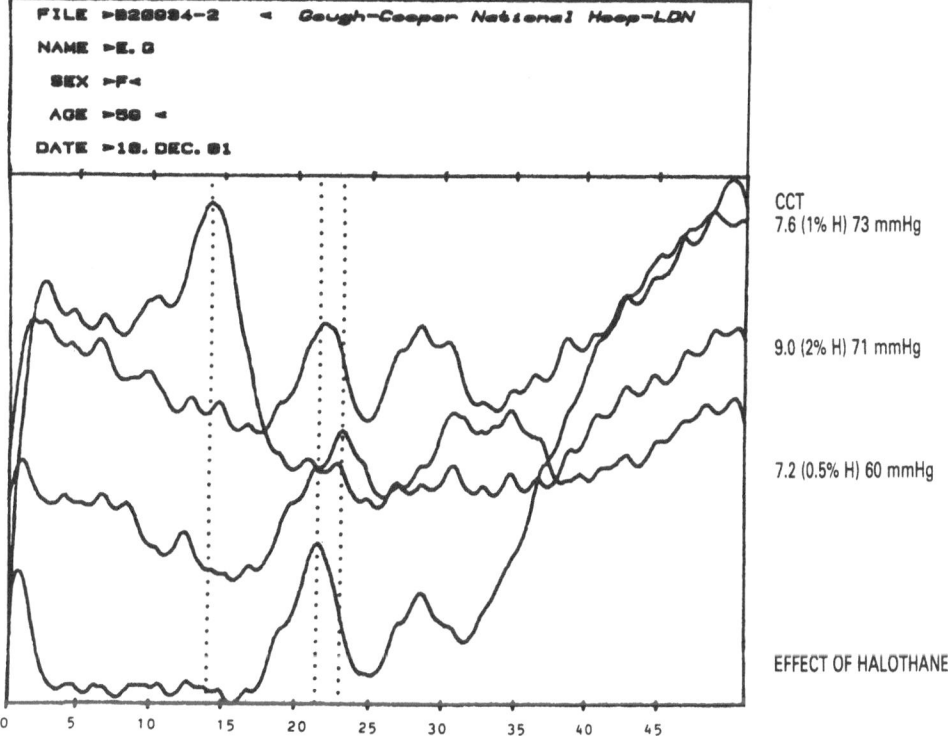

Fig. 4b. CCT change after change of halothane concentration. Another
          case. CCT increased from 7.6 msec to 9.0 msec when halo-
          thane increased from 1% to 2% and returned to 7.2 msec when
          halothane was reduced to 0.5%.

flap, opening of the dura and dissection of the vessels was without significant change in CCT but brain retraction was found to create an interhemispheric difference, more than 0.6 msecs in four patients, the retracted hemisphere showing the longer conduction time. (Figure 5a and b).

A significant increase in CCT was found in 11 of 15 patients immediately after the application of a clip to the aneurysm neck, the prolongation ranging from 0.4 to 3 msecs. The mean CCT after clip was 8.1 ± 1.5 msecs, preclip CCT being 7.1 ± 0.7 msecs (p<0.05).

The technique has proven of value in the assessment of the safety or otherwise of the application of temporary clips. Temporary clips have been applied to major vessels, (terminal carotid or middle cerebral artery) in 8 patients during operation. The duration of clip has varied from 1-13 minutes. In five cases there was no detectable change in CCT despite clipping the terminal carotid or proximal middle cerebral artery, although a reduction of amplitude of the N20 peak was invariably noticed. In the others, CCT was

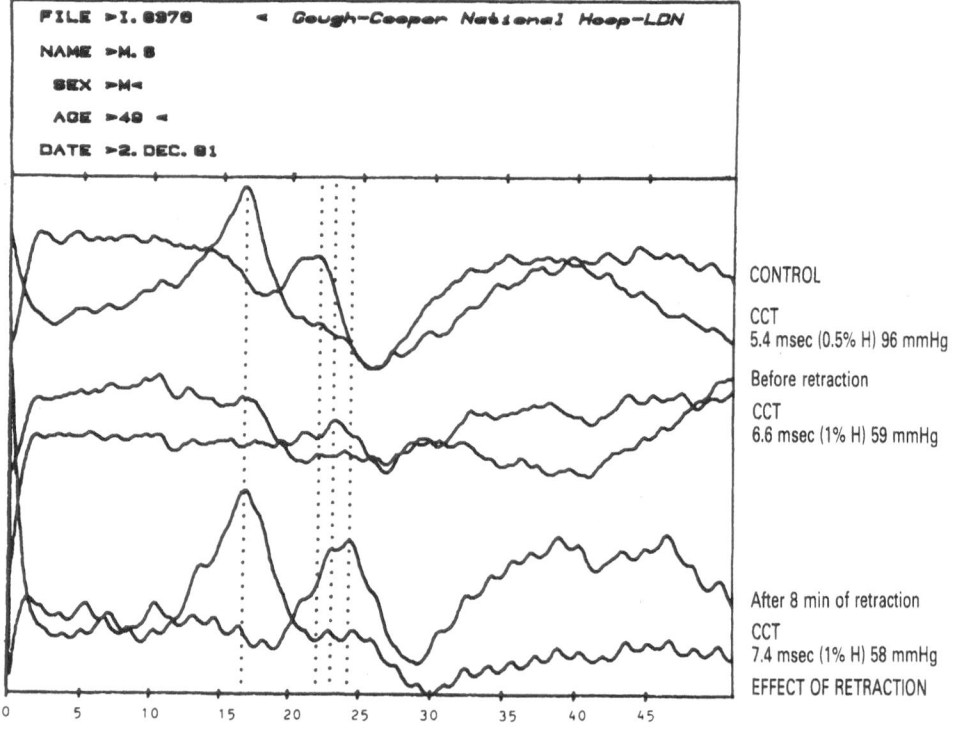

Fig. 5a. Shows that brain retraction created a prolongation of CCT on operated hemisphere from 6.6 msec to 7.4 msec (5a), with a 1.6 msec interhemispheric difference (5b).

prolonged, but in each case it returned to the preclip level in 15-20 minutes (Figure 6). In one instance (Figure 7) CCT remained prolonged and amplitude much diminished after the application of a clip to the neck of a middle cerebral artery aneurysm, and further dissection revealed that an unsuspected hidden opercularbranch had been included in the clip. CCT and amplitudes returned to normal when the clip was repositioned. In only one case has significant neurological deficit been related to preoperative CCT recording, a giant ophthalmic artery aneurysm whose CCT rose to over 10 msecs on application of a terminal carotid intracranial clip, and a clip to the internal carotid artery in the neck. This patient had a significant central hemispheral deficit with mutism and fluctuating bilateral signs for some weeks postoperatively, but eventually made a good recovery, the CCT returning to normal within half an hour of removal of the temporary clips, and fluctuating thereafter in relation to the neurological deficit.

In uncomplicated cases, CCT was usually slightly prolonged at the end of surgery (6.8 ± 0.6 msecs), significantly higher than the

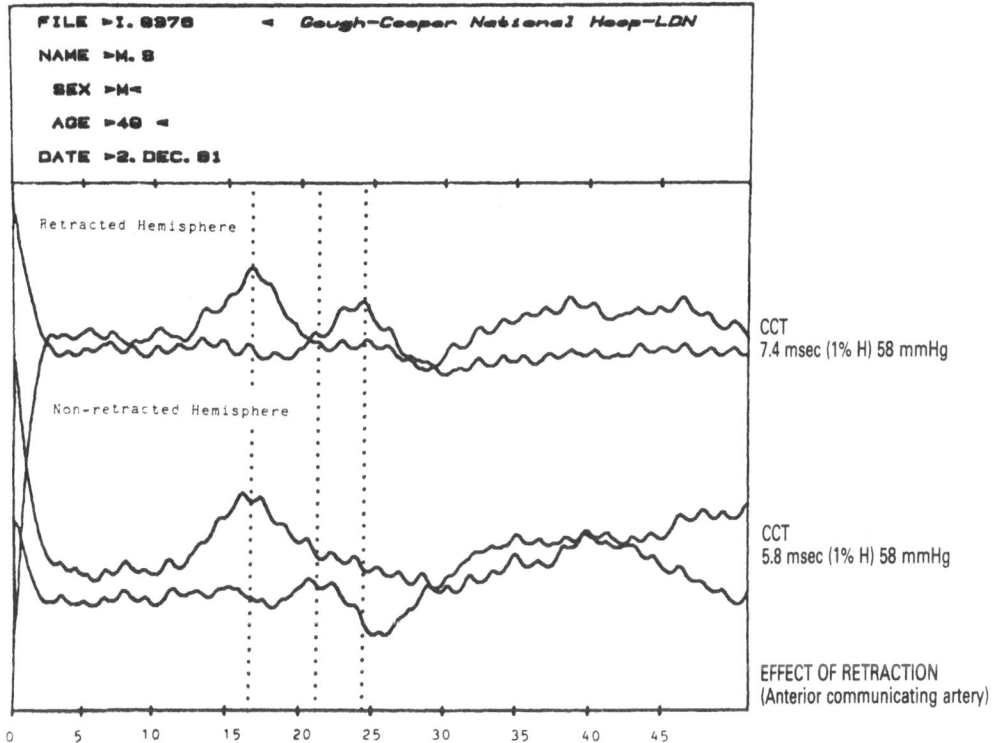

Fig. 5b. Shows that brain retraction created a prolongation of CCT on operated hemisphere from 6.6 msec to 7.4 msec (5a), with a 1.6 msec interhemisphere difference (5b).

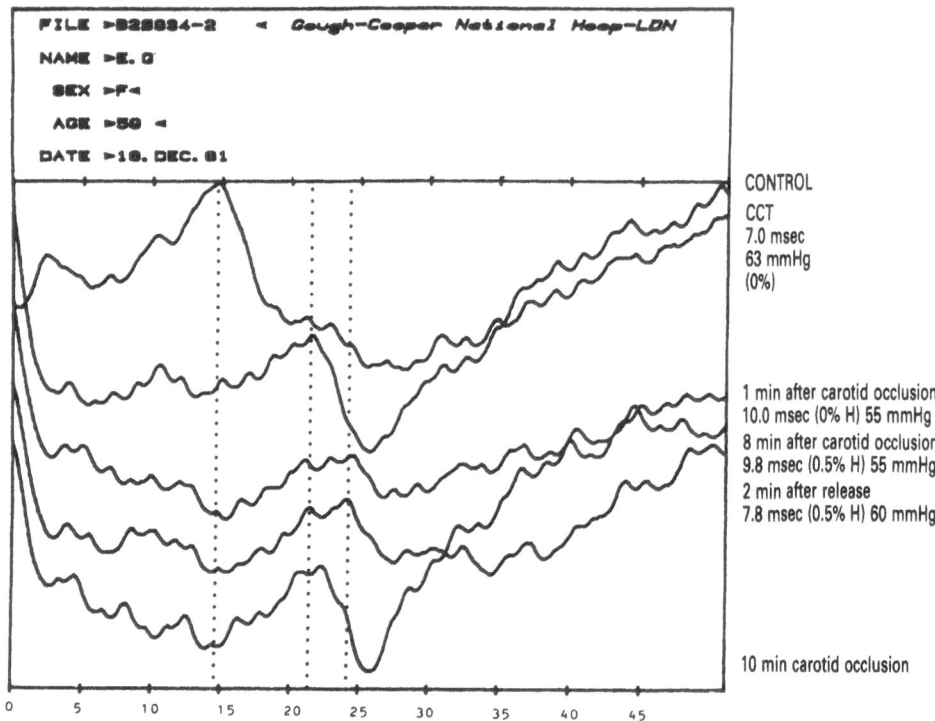

Fig. 6.   Patient EG had a terminal carotid ophthalmic artery giant
          aneurysm.   During surgery carotid artery was occluded tem-
          porarly.   CCT increased to 10.0 msec from 7.0 msec after
          clipping, reduced to 7.8 msec 9 minutes after restored
          circulation.

preoperative level, but not different from the value under the induction of anaesthesia.   In all cases, CCT shortened to a level approximately the same as preoperative level on return of consciousness in
the recovery room, provided the patient was without neurological
deficit.

DISCUSSION

     We have felt the N14-N20 interval represents conduction time
within the central nervous system, N14 taking its origin from the
dorsal column nuclei, and N20 probably from the cortex (6, 3).   Our
animal experimentation has confirmed N20 as most likely based in
cortex.

     Lengthening of CCT has frequently served as a premonitor of
clinical deterioration, although exceptions certainly do exist, and
it appears that significant prolongation of CCT in the preoperative

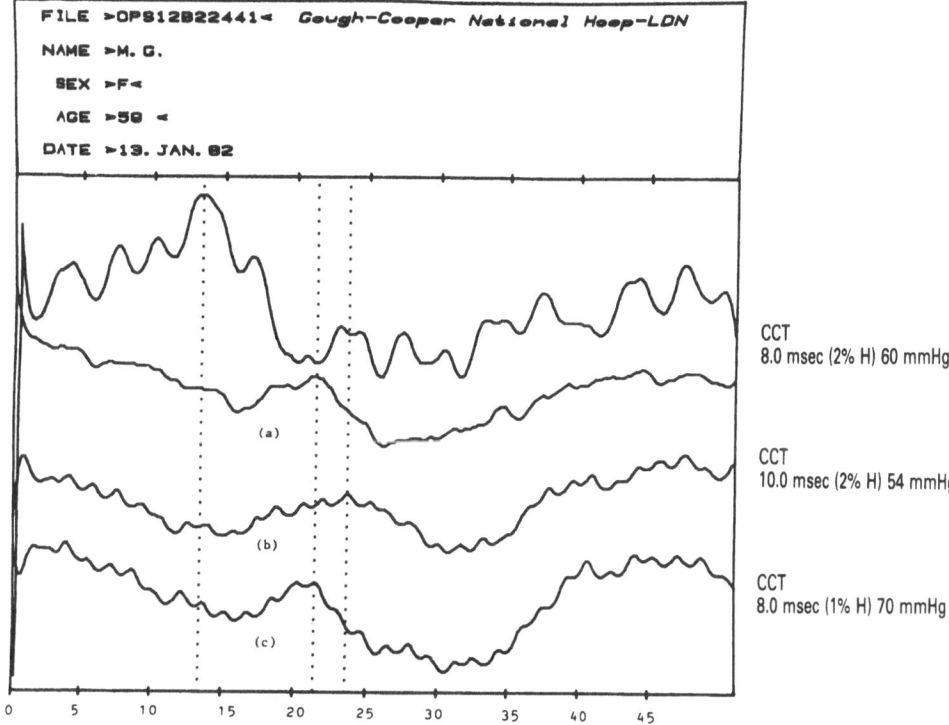

Fig. 7.   Patient MG had a SAH from a right middle cerebral artery
          aneurysm. Pre-clip tracing (a) showed CCT 8.0 msec, after
          clipping (b) CCT prolonged to 10 msec and with a low ampli-
          tude. One opercular branch was found to be in the clip; 15
          minutes after repositioning of clip CCT reduced to 8.0 msec
          with a better cortical peak (c).

phase probably indicates a hemispheral deficit in blood flow.   In
grade 3 cases this has been sufficient now to persuade us to postpone
surgery.   There is a significant difference between CCT in grade 4
patients, considered as a group and compared with controls, and we
have found that significant prolongation of CCT into the second
postoperative week can be significantly correlated with the poor
outcome at two months.   Our preoperative studies suggest that the
induction of halothane anaesthesia, the development of significant
hypotension, or the application of a clip to the aneurysm, may all be
expected to prolong CCT significantly, but from the few cases in the
present series where significant neurological deficit has appeared
postoperatively, it seems that a conduction time of up to 10 msecs
during operation is without necessary sequela, and provided the CCT
has returned to approximately induction levels by the close of surgery, all may be well.

REFERENCES

Allison, T., and Hume, A. L., 1981, A comparative analysis of short
    latency somatosensory evoked potentials in man, monkey, cat
    and rat, Exp.Neurol., 72:592-611.
Branston, N. M., and Symon, L., 1980, Cortical EP, blood flow and
    potassium changes in experimental ischaemia, in "Evoked Pot-
    entials," C. Barber ed., MTP Lancaster, 527-530.
Branston, N. M., Symon, L., Crockard, H. A., and Pasztor, E., 1974,
    Relationship between the cortical evoked potential and local
    cortical blood flow following acute middle cerebral artery
    occlusion in the baboon, Exp.Neurol., 45:195-208.
Chiappa, K. M., Clevi, S. K., and Young, R. R., 1980, Short latency
    SEPs following median nerve stimulation in patients with
    neurological lesions, in: "Prog.Clin.Neurophysiol., J. E.
    Desmedt, ed., Karger, Basle, 57-68.
Desmedt, J. E., and Cheron, G., 1980, Central somatosensory con-
    duction in man: neural generators and interpeak latencies of
    the far field components recorded from neck and right or left
    scalp and earlobes, Electroencephal.Clin.Neurophysiol.,
    50:382-403.
Hargadine, J. R., Branston N. M., and Symon, L., 1980, Central con-
    duction time in primate brain ischemia - a study in baboons,
    Stroke, 11(6):637-642.
Hume, A. L., and Cant, B. R., 1978, Conduction time in central
    somato-sensory pathways in man, Electroencephal.Clin.Neuro-
    physiol., 45:361-375.
Jones, S. J., 1977, Shunt latency potentials recorded from the neck
    and scalp following median nerve stimulation in man, Electro-
    encephal.Clin.Neurophysiol., 43:853-863.
El Negamy, E., and Sedgewick, M., 1978, Properties of a spinal soma-
    tosensory evoked potential recorded in man, J.Neurol.Neuro-
    surg. and Psychiat., 41:762-781.
El Negamy, E., and Sedgewick, M., 1979, Delayed cervical somatosen-
    sory potentials in cervical spondylosis, J.Neurol.Neurosurg.
    and Psychiat., 42:238-241.
Small, D. G., Beauchamp, M., and Matthews, W. B., 1980, Subcortical
    somatosensory evoked potentials in normal man and patients
    with CNS lesions, in: "Prog.Clin.Neurophysiol," J. E. Desmedt,
    ed., Karger, Basle, 190-204.
Symon, L., Hargadine, J., Zawirski, M., and N. M. Branston, 1979,
    Central conduction time as an index of ischaemia in subarach-
    noid haemorrhage, J.Neurol.Sci., 44:95-103.
Trojaborg, W., and Boysen, G., 1973, Relationship between EEG, re-
    gional cerebral blood flow and internal carotid artery pres-
    sure during carotid endarterectomy, Electroencephal.Clin.
    Neurophysiol., 34:1-9.

RECENT ASPECTS OF HYPOTENSIVE DRUG

EFFECTS ON INTRACRANIAL PRESSURE

V. W. A. Pickerodt

Dept. of Anaesthesia
Ev. Waldkrankenhaus
Berlin-Spandau, FRG

Increases in intracranial pressure (ICP) induced by pharmacological agents used for lowering arterial blood pressure may have
serious effects on the brain particularly in the presence of a space-
occupying lesion (SOL): a reduction of the cerebral perfusion pressure (CPP) may compromise cerebral perfusion and the occurrence of
pressure gradients within the skull may lead to brain shifts with
subsequent herniation at the tentorium.

The effects of volatile anaesthetic agents on ICP have been
convincingly demonstrated in numerous publications particularly by
McDowall and coworkers. However, enflurane has only recently been
recommended as the agent of choice for controlled hypotension in
neurosurgical patients (FIRN, 1981).

Apart from the volatile anaesthetic agents and the unacceptable
technique of hemorrhagic hypotension the interest is focussed on
three substances which are used alone or in various combinations:
trimetaphan (TMP), sodium nitroprusside (SNP) and trinitroglycerine
(TNG). Trimetaphan has been used routinely for the induction of
hypotension long before the other two agents. The effects of TMP on
ICP have been investigated by Stullken and Sokoll (1975) who reported
a significant increase in ICP (4 mmHg) at an arterial blood pressure
of 40 mmHg whereas Turner et al. (1977) did not find a significant
change in ICP in a group of 21 patients receiving trimetaphan.
However, 16 of the 21 patients exhibited an increase in ICP but
this increase was small except in two patients. In one of the two
patients ICP continued to rise to 45 mmHg after the cessation of
trimetaphan infusion and that points to the importance of the posthypotensive period when in cases of disturbed autoregulation ICP may
follow the arterial blood pressure. These authors also mentioned the

145

importance of the rapidity of blood pressure changes which has later been confirmed by Marsh and coworkers, 1979. More recently, Larsen et al., 1980 demonstrated a decrease in ICP associated with trimeta-phan hypotension.

Turner and coauthors 1975, 1977 described the effects of SNP on ICP. Their results obtained from patients mainly with cerebral tumors demonstrated an increase in ICP when the blood pressure was lowered with SNP to 90 and 80% of the baseline blood pressure but ICP returned to its starting value when BP reached 70% of control. Similar results have been obtained in hyperventilated patients but the increase in ICP did not reach the level of significance. Inter-estingly the baseline ICP of the hyperventilated patients was higher than that of normoventilated patients.

Larsen et al. (1980) confirmed these findings in animal exper-iments showing the highest ICP values in the recovery period of the arterial blood corresponding with the record of one of the patients described by Turner et al. (1977) where a recovery of blood pressure led to a further marked increase in ICP. The results of Cottrell et al. (1978) vary from Turners in so far as the baseline ICP was much higher and continued to rise when the blood pressure was reduced to 70% of control.

Trinitroglycerin (TNG) is the oldest substance in clinical use but the last to be introduced in the practice of intraoperative controlled hypotension. Chestnut and coworkers (1978) evaluated the use of intravenous nitroglycerin for neurosurgical patients and considered TNG as the "agent of choice for the production of con-trolled hypotension during neurosurgery". However these authors did not record ICP in their patients. Work by Gupta and Cottrell (1980), Rogers et al. (1979) and a case report by Gagnon et al. (1979) demon-strated significant increases in ICP associated with nitroglycerin-induced hypotension. In contrast, Burt and coauthors (1981) showed a decrease in ICP in dogs with a space-occupying lesion when a bolus injection of TNG reduced the blood pressure below 75% of control. Dohi, Matsumoto and Takahashi (1981) using bolus injections of TNG in awake and anaesthetized humans found increases in CSF pressure which were significant though transient.

In a series of animal experiments we infused nitroglycerin to cats anaesthetized with pentobarbitone, intubated and artificially ventilated with 66% Nitrous oxide in oxygen, muscular relaxation being achieved with alcuronium. In all experiments ICP was recorded via a needle in the posterior fossa. In one group of animals a small supratentorial epidural balloon serving as an artificial space-occu-pying lesion (SOL) was slowly inflated to produce an increase in ICP to 15 mmHg.

Figure 1: TNG was continuously given to three groups of cats via a central venous catheter (group I = normoventilated, Pa_{CO_2}: 31,

Group	n	Technique of hypotension	
I	23	TNG (Normoventilation)	●——●
II	30	TNG (Hyperventilation)	▲——▲
III	47	TNG (SOL , Normoventilation)	■——■
IV	12	SNP (Normoventilation)	○——○

Fig. 1

63 mm Hg, group II = hyperventilated, Pa_{CO_2}: 19, 85 mmHg, group III = normoventilated with SOL, Pa_{CO_2}: 32, 42 mmHg) and the effects were compared with a group of normoventilated cats (group IV, Pa_{CO_2}: 30, 86 mmHg) receiving sodium nitroprusside (SNP). ECG, instantaneous heart rate (HR), arterial blood pressure (BP), ICP and central venous pressure was continuously recorded. Figure 2 illustrates the effects of an infusion of 0.25 mg/min TNG (= 83 µg/kg/min) in a group I animal. Almost no change in heart rate occurred whereas mean arterial pressure (MAP) decreased from 140 mmHg to 108 mmHg and mean ICP increased by 5.3 mmHg. Only minor changes in CVP were seen in this experiment.

In order to compare the effects on ICP for a given blood pressure reduction, the change in ICP (Δ ICP) was plotted against mean arterial pressure (% MAP) (Figure 3). In the three groups of animals without intracranial pathology, ICP increased moderately; whereas in the animals with SOL, ICP increased considerably. A more detailed analysis of the experiments with SOL revealed remarkably different types of ICP changes: Figure 4 presents the normal response with an increase in ICP during reduction of blood pressure and the return of BP and ICP towards control levels. In contrast, Figure 5 shows a secondary ICP increase in the period of recovering blood pressure suggesting impairment of autoregulation. The same type of reaction has been shown to occur with halothane-induced hypotension by Keaney et al., (1973) and with SNP (Turner et al., 1975).

As TNG was administered repeatedly to each animal with at least 30 min between each hypotensive period, eventually every animal with SOL showed dilatation of one or both pupils during the TNG-induced hypotensive phase. In a further 8 experiments the pupils were

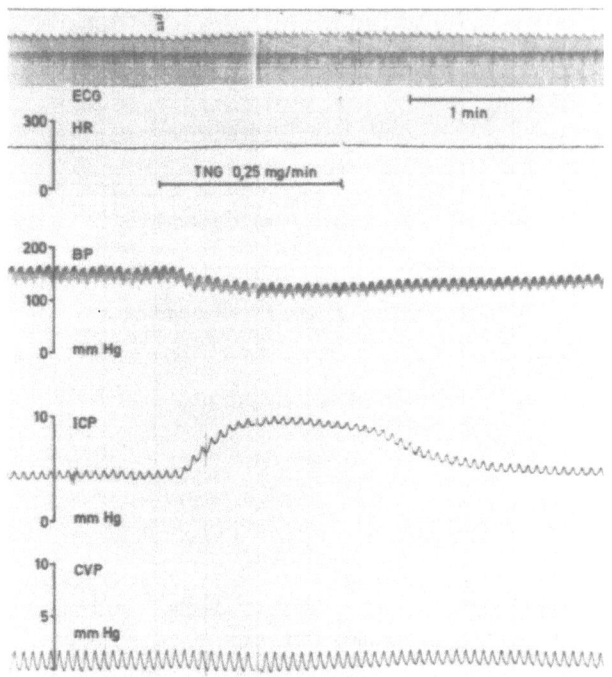

Fig. 2

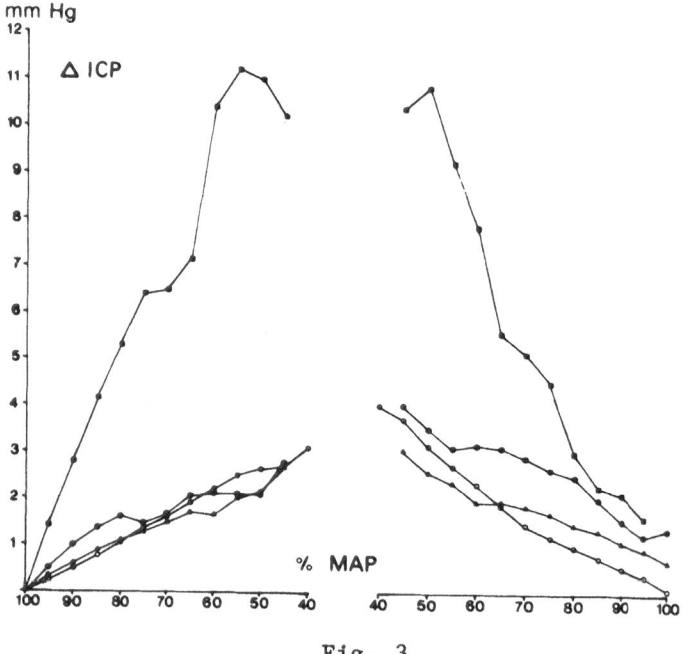

Fig. 3

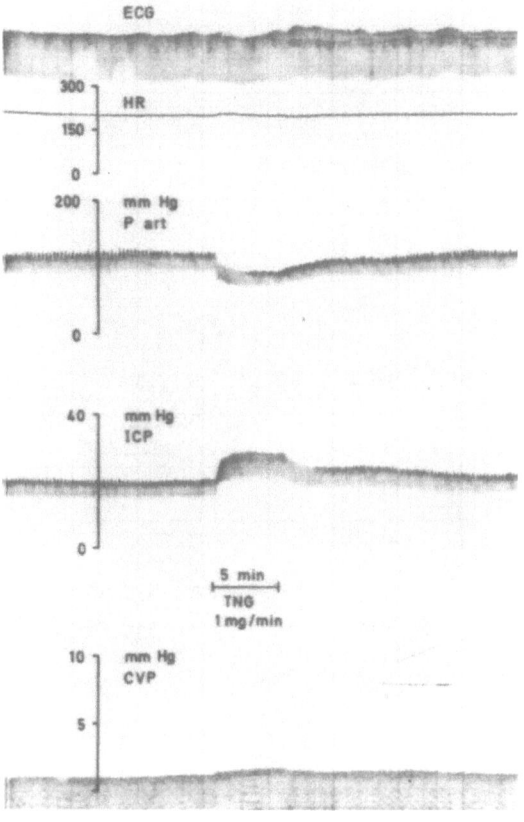

Fig. 4

already dilated before the onset of hypotension. Accordingly group
III was subdivided into three subgroups (Figure 6).

Figure 7 shows mean values of MAP and ICP during TNC administration and in the five posthypotensive minutes (group IIIa, b and c).
MAP in group IIIb is significantly below MAP of group IIIa animals
and ICP returns towards control in group IIIa but remains significantly elevated in group IIIb, indicating loss of autoregulation.

Calculated cerebral perfusion pressure (CPP = MAP - ICP) in the
experiments (Figure 8) with pupillary dilatation (IIIb) was significantly less than CPP of the animals without signs of brainstem herniation.

The likely existence of a pressure gradient across the tentorium
which has been demonstrated by Fitch and McDowall (1971) in similar
experiments during the administration of halothane may have even
further compromised cerebral supratentorial perfusion and caused

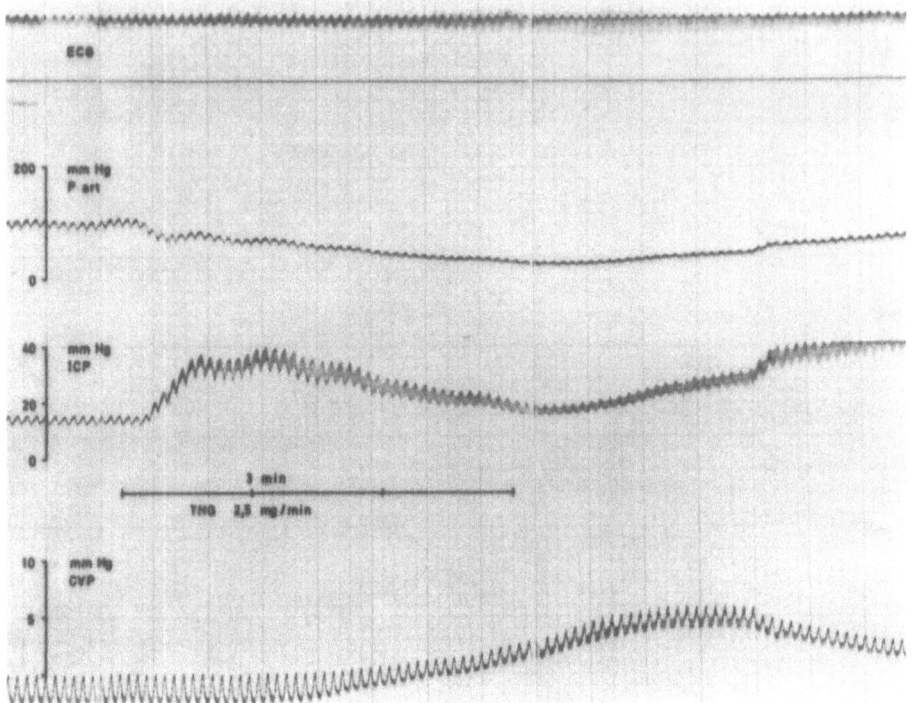

Fig. 5

Group	n		
III	47	SOL (Normoventilation)	
III a	31	SOL (pupils normal)	■——■
III b	8	SOL (pupils dilated during hypotension)	●——●
III c	8	SOL (pupils dilated befor hypotension)	▲——▲

Fig. 6

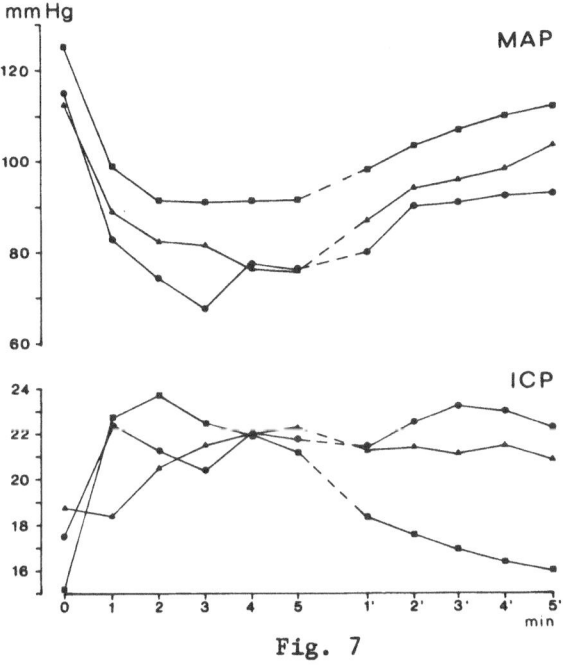

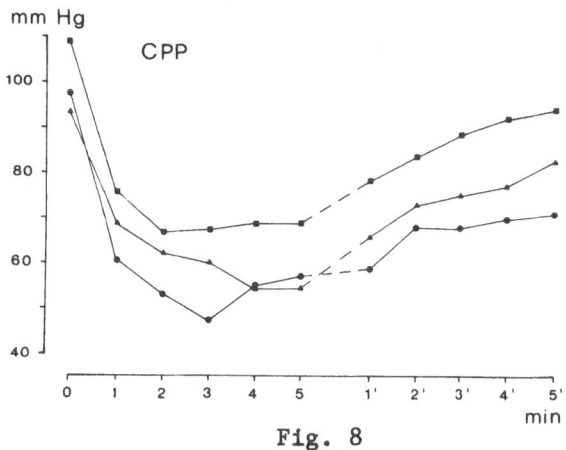

Fig. 7

Fig. 8

cerebral vasoparalysis. Once vasoparalysis has occurred, ICP may
decrease with reduction of arterial pressure: this was observed in
four experiments and may explain the conflicting results reported in
the literature.

From the experimental results it is concluded:

1. In animals without intracranial pathology cerebral vasodilating agents such as sodium nitroprusside or nitroglycerin produce a small though significant increase of ICP.
2. Prior hyperventilation does not modify this response.
3. In experiments with artificial supratentorial space-occupying lesions ICP increases markedly.
4. In these animals ICP remained increased during the recovery of the arterial pressure, indicating loss of autoregulation.
5. Brainstem herniation, indicated by pupillary dilatation may occur during the administration of TNG.

REFERENCES

Burt, D. E. R., Verniquet, A. J. W., and Homi, J., 1981, Effects of nitroglycerin-induced hypotension on intracranial pressure in dogs, Br.J.Anaesth., 53:186P.
Chestnut, J. S., Albin, M. S., Gonzales-Abola, E., Newfield, P., and Maroon, J. C., 1978, Clinical evaluation of intravenous nitroglycerin for neurosurgery, J.Neurosurg., 48:704.
Cottrell, J. E., Patel, K., Turndorf, H., and Ransohoff, J., 1978, Intracranial pressure changes induced by sodium nitroprusside in patients with intracranial mass lesions, J.Neurosurg., 48:329.
Dohi, S., Matsumoto, M., and Takahashi, T., 1981, The effects of nitroglycerin on cerebrospinal fluid pressure in awake and anesthetized humans, Anesthesiology, 54:511.
Firn, S., 1981, Enflurane for controlled hypotension, Proc. Zentraleuropäischer Anaesthesiekongress, Berlin, p.169.
Fitch, W., and McDowall, D. G., 1971, The effect of halothane on intracranial pressure gradients in the presence of intracranial space-occupying lesions, Br.J.Anaesth., 43:904.
Gagnon, R. L., Marsh, M. L., SMith, R. W., and Shapiro, H. M., 1979, Intracranial hypertension caused by nitroglycerin, Anesthesiology, 51:86.
Gupta, B., and Cottrell, J. E., 1980, Nitroprusside and nitroglycerin induced intracranial pressure changes, in: "Intracranial Pressure IV," K. Shulman, A. Marmarou, J. D. Miller, D. P. Becker, G. M. Hochwald, and M. Brock, eds., Springer Verlag, Berlin-Heidelberg-New York, p.613.
Keaney, N. P., Pickerodt, V. W., McDowall, D. G., Coroneos, N. J., Turner, J. M., and Shah, Z. P., 1978, Cerebral circulatory and metabolic effects of hypotension produced by deep halothane anaesthesia, J.Neurol.Neurosurg.Psychiat., 36:898.
Larsen, R., Teichmann, J., Schenk, D.-D., Radke, J., Drobnik, L., and Kettler, D., 1980, Kontrollierte Hypotension: Der Einfluss von Halothan, Nitroprussid-Natrium und Trimetaphan auf Hirndurchblutung, Hirndruck und Hirnmetabolismus, in:

"Anaesthesiology and Intensive Care Medicine," K. H. Weis, and
G. Cunitz, eds., 25 Jahre DGAI, Springer-Verlag Berlin-
Heidelberg New York, p.469.

Marsh, M. L., Aidinis, S. J., Naughton, K. V. H., Marshall, L. F.,
and Shapiro, H. M., 1979, The technique of nitroprusside
administration modifies the intracranial pressure response,
Anesthesiology, 51:538.

Rogers, M. C., Hamburger, C., Owen, K., and Epstein, M. H., 1979,
Intracranial pressure in the cat during nitroglycerin-induced
hypotension, Anesthesiology, 51:227.

Stullken, E. H., and Sokoll, M. D., 1975, Intracranial pressure
during hypotension and subsequent vasopressor therapy in
anesthetized cats, Anesthesiology, 42:425.

Turner, J. M., Powell, D., Gibson, R. M., and McDowall, D. G., 1975,
The effects of sodium nitroprusside on intracranial pressure
and autoregulation, in: "Intracranial Pressure II", N.
Lundberg, U. Ponten, and M. Brock, eds., Springer-Verlag,
Berlin-Heidelberg-New York, p.345.

Turner, J. M., Powell, D., Gibson, R. M., and McDowall, D. G., 1977,
Intracranial pressure changes in neurosurgical patients during
hypotension induced with sodium nitroprusside or trimetaphan,
Br.J.Anaesth., 49:419.

IV

MORPHOLOGICAL ASPECTS OF CONTROLLED HYPOTENSION

THE NEUROPATHOLOGY OF STAGNANT HYPOXIA

D. I. Graham

University Department of Neuropathology
Institute of Neurological Sciences
Southern General Hospital, Glasgow, Scotland

INTRODUCTION

Hypoxic brain damage may occur in any situation where there is an inadequate supply of oxygen to nerve cells It is therefore a potential hazard to any patient subjected to general anaesthesia, a severe episode of hypotension, cardiac arrest, status epilepticus and carbon monoxide intoxication. The eventual degree of clinical recovery will be determined by whether or not satisfactory resuscitation can be achieved before permanent brain damage ensues. Crises of this kind are not uncommon in clinical practice but the central question as to what duration of hypoxia defines the watershed between recovery of the tissues and extensive permanent injury has not been critically defined in man (Plum, 1973). The reasons for this include the lack of precise physiological data about the patients' cardiovascular and respiratory status at the time of crisis since the immediate priority is resuscitation, and therefore such basic information as the precise duration of the cardiac arrest or blood pressure and heart rate during severe hypotension is very rarely available. In such cases the neuropathological descriptions, however exhaustive, may well explain the final neuropsychiatric status of the patient but can at best indicate only tentatively the nature of the episode itself.

Matters are further complicated by the fact that post mortem examination of patients with severe hypoxic brain damage are usually carried out under warrant by the forensic pathologist, who often feels obliged to slice the unfixed brain in the mortuary. In these conditions it is impossible to recognize recent hypoxic brain damage even when subsequent histological examination shows severe and extensive neuronal necrosis (Graham, 1977). When the brain has been

properly dissected after adequate (up to 3 weeks immersion in
buffered 10% formol saline), focal hypoxic brain damage of about
18-24 hours duration may just be recognizable but even an experienced
neuropathologist may fail to identify diffuse hypoxic brain damage if
it is less than some 3-4 days duration. The extent and severity of
hypoxic brain damage can be identified and its distribution analyzed
only by the microscopic examination of many large bilateral and
representative sections of the brain. It is, however, often possible
to establish that a patient has suffered hypoxic brain damage on the
basis of a more restricted examination provided the pathologist knows
that certain areas of the brain are selectively vulnerable and is
familiar with the cytological and histological appearances of ischaemic nerve cell change (Brierly, 1976., Brown, 1977).

     The identification of specific changes in nerve cells is made
difficult in the human brain because of the frequent occurrence of
histological artefacts. They are due partly to post mortem handling
and to the slow penetration of fixative. Studies in experimental
animals and in selected human material have shown that there is an
identifiable process, namely ischaemic nerve cell change, which is
considered to be the neuropathological common denominator in all
types of hypoxia in which circulation is either sustained partially
via collateral arteries or restored after a period of absolute ischaemia (Brierley, 1976; Brown, 1977; Garcia et al., 1977). More
recently a further type of ischaemic nerve cell injury has been
reported to occur in different forms of permanent, complete ischaemia
(Arsenio-Nunes et al., 1973; Kalimo et al., 1977; Jenkins et al.,
1979a) but the significance of this remains uncertain and controversial (Agardh et al., 1981; Brierley and Brown, 1981).

     It is not the intention to review all aspects of the pathology
of hypoxic brain damage, but rather to concentrate on the main patterns of stagnant hypoxic damage that follow a global reduction in
the supply of blood to the brain in both man and the experimental
animal. There are two main types, viz. ischaemic in which there is a
global arrest of cerebral blood flow, and oligaemic in which there is
a global reduction in blood supply.

STAGNANT HYPOXIC BRAIN DAMAGE IN MAN

Ischaemic

     A global arrest of blood flow to the brain is most commonly the
result of cardiac arrest. This is usually a complication of some
surgical procedure under general anaethesia. If death occurs within
24-36 hours of the arrest, the brain may appear normal externally and
on section (Figure 1). Microscopy, however reveals diffuse neuronal
necrosis with a characteristic pattern of selective vulnerability.
Thus the hypoxic brain damage is commonly greater within sulci than

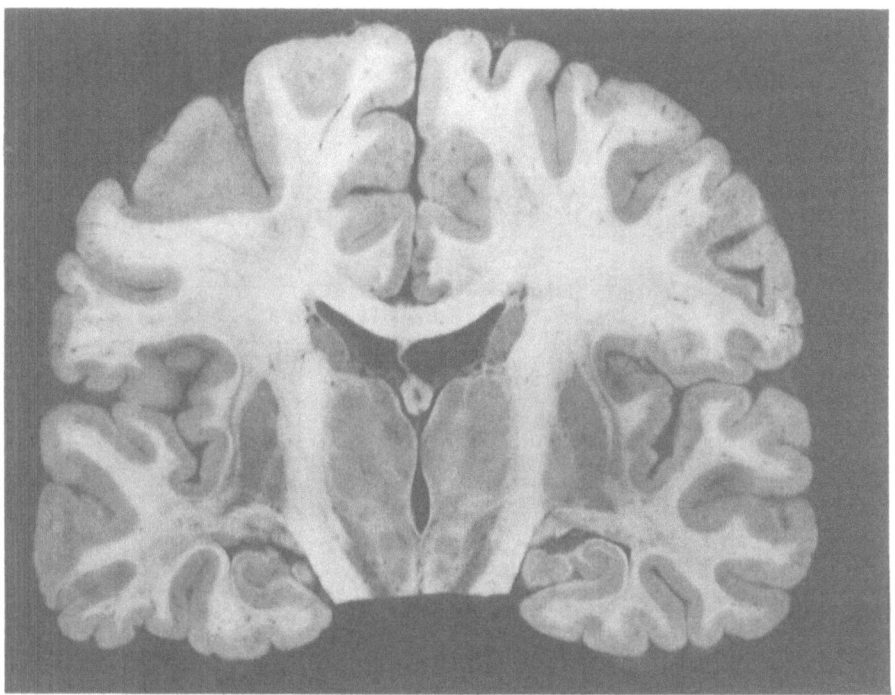

Fig. 1.   Coronal section of brain from patient who survived 48 hours
           after cardiac arrest.   There are no macroscopic abnormal-
           ities.   (Reproduced by kind permission of the Editor of the
           British Medical Journal from Graham, J.Clin.Path., 30,
           Suppl. (Roy.Coll.Path), 11:170-180.)

at the crests of gyri and is maximal in the third, fifth and sixth
layers of the cortex (Figure 2) in the posterior halves of the
cerebral hemispheres.   In the Ammon's horn, the Sommer sector
(Figures 3a and b) and endfolium are the most vulnerable.   The pattern of damage in the basal ganglia is less constant.   Hypoxic damage
in the thalamus is most common in the anterior, dorso-medial and
ventro-lateral nuclei.   In the cerebellum there is characteristically
diffuse necrosis of Purkinje cells.   Damage to the brain stem nuclei
tends to be more severe in infants and young children than in adults.

    Patients with diffuse brain damage due to cardiac arrest rarely
survive for more than a few days but occasionally they may remain
alive in a vegetative state (Jennett and Plum, 1972).   With increasing survival the necrotic tissue is usually replaced by a glio-
mesodermal scar.   When this occurs there may be an appreciable reduction in the weight of the brain, evidence of marked atrophy in the
selectively vulnerable areas and considerable enlargement of the
ventricles (Figure 4).

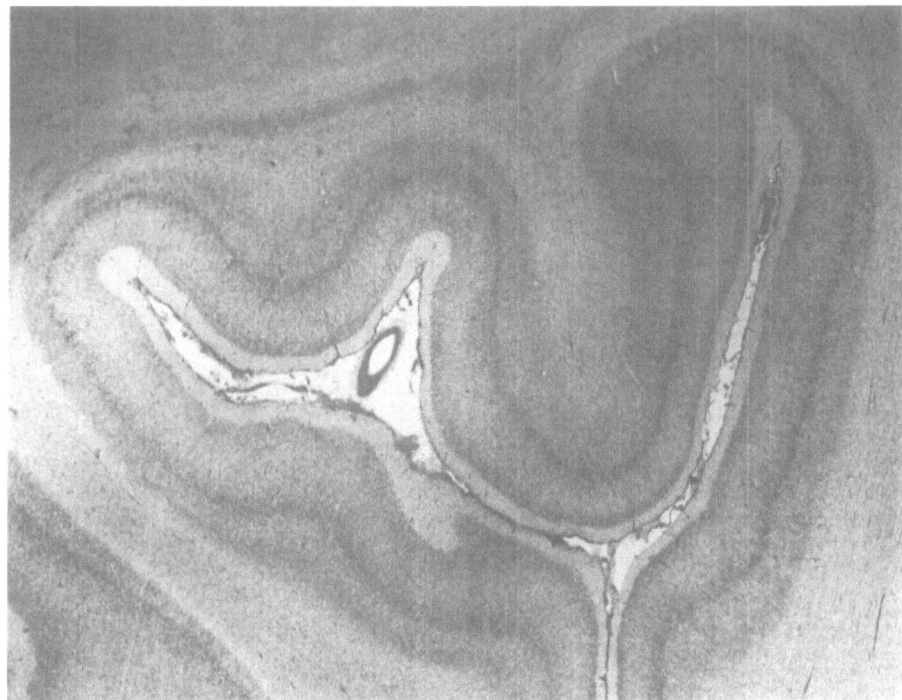

Fig. 2.   Same patient as Figure 1.   Note subtotal (laminar) necrosis
of the third, fifth and sixth cortical layers with relative
sparing of the second and fourth layers (darker staining).
Cresyl violet x 3.2.

Oligaemic

Brain perfusion pressure can fall to about 50 mm Hg without
a significant reduction in cerebral blood flow (CBF).   Below this
figure the capacity for the autoregulation of blood flow is lost and
flow is then pressure dependent so that if perfusion pressure con-
tinues to fall, CBF will be reduced to a level at which the EEG
declines and eventually becomes isoelectric, and if this state persists long enough brain damage will occur.

On the basis of evidence and experimental studies on primates,
brain damage due to oligaemia appears to be caused by a major and
abrupt episode of hypotension followed by a rapid return to a normal
blood pressure.   It is often seen after a conscious patient has
collapsed as a result of a sudden reduction in cardiac output, viz.
due to ischaemic heart disease (Adams et al., 1966), and may occur
after carotid artery occlusion (Romanoul and Abramowicz, 1964) and in
the anaesthetized subject during dental procedures (Brierley and
Miller, 1966),particularly in the sitting position.   More recently it

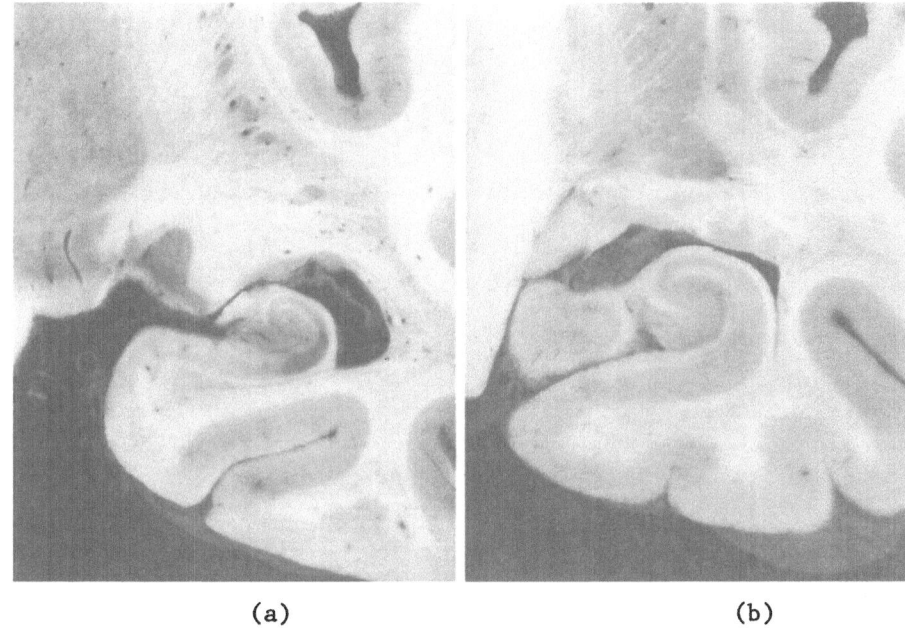

(a)   (b)

Fig. 3.   (a) Normal right Ammon's horn to compare with Figure 3(b).
           (b) Right Ammon's horn.   There is necrosis of the Sommer
           sector.   (Both reproduced by kind permission of the Editor
           of the British Medical Journal from Graham, J.Clin.Path.,
           30, Suppl. (Roy.Coll.Path), 11:170-180.

has been described following the use of methlmethacrylic bone cement
(Adams et al., 1972), in patients undergoing emergency treatment with
antihypertensive agents (Graham, 1975), and in patients dying from
non-missile head injuries (Graham et al., 1978).   Because of the
precipitate decrease in arterial pressure there is a transient failure of autoregulation and a severe reduction in CBF in the regions
most removed from the parent arterial stems, that is, the boundary
zones between the arterial territories of the cortex of the cerebral
and cerebellar hemispheres (Figure 5).   The resulting lesions vary in
size, are usually asymmetrical and may be unilateral.   There is
variable involvement of the basal ganglia.   The Ammon's horn and
brain stem are usually not involved.

STAGNANT HYPOXIC BRAIN DAMAGE IN THE EXPERIMENTAL ANIMAL

Ischaemic

     Complete arrest of the cerebral circulation in the experimental
animal is difficult to achieve largely because of the brain's extensive protective collateral circulation.   While the blood flow through

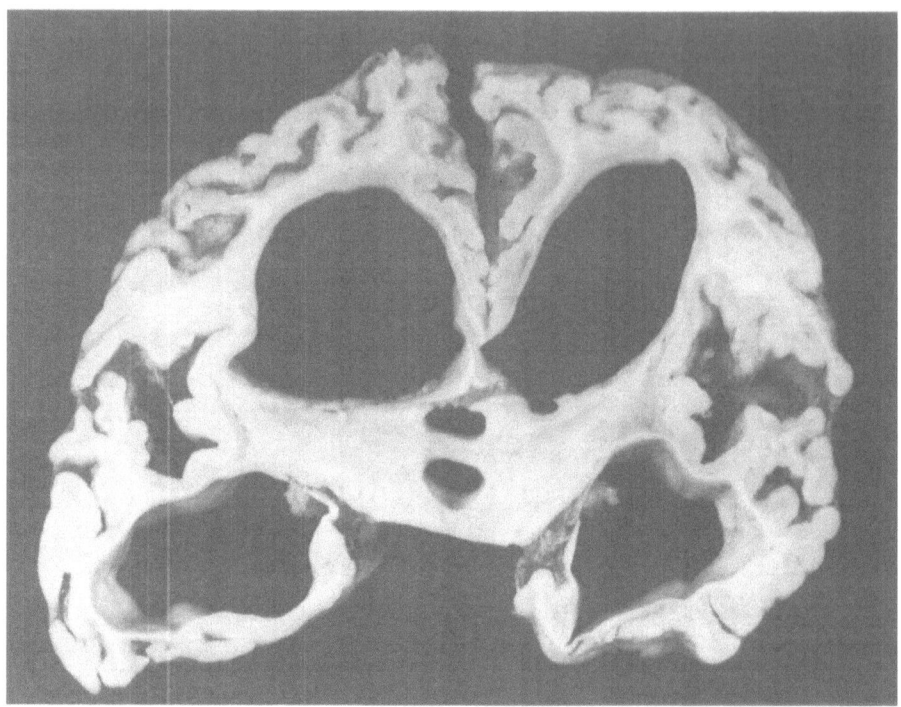

Fig. 4.   Coronal section of brain from patient who survived for four
           years in a vegetative state after cardiac arrest. The
           cortex is greatly narrowed and there is gross essentially
           symmetrical enlargement of the ventricles. The Ammon's
           horns and the thalami are also small. (Reproduced by kind
           permission of the Editor of the British Medical Journal from
           Graham, J.Clin.Path., 30, Suppl.(Roy.Coll.Path), 11:170-180.

the carotid and vertebral arteries has been arrested by a variety of
techniques, it has proved much more difficult to eliminate potential
inflow from arteries in the spinal canal. Methods to circumvent this
collateral blood supply to the brain have included the division of
the vessels at an earlier operation (Patterson et al., 1968; Jenkins
et al., 1979b) and the induction of hypotension after occluding the
major arteries in the neck (Nemoto et al., 1977). Cardiac arrest
induced by an AC fibrillator (Lin et al., 1979) and cross tracheal
clamping (Hendrickx et al., 1981) have also been investigated. In
spite of meticulous technique, however, there must remain some uncer-
tainty as to whether complete cerebral circulatory arrest has been
attained in these experiments. The only models therefore that exclude any collateral circulation and ensure a square wave cessation
and restoration of blood flow to the brain are those employing an
isolated perfused head through which circulatory arrest is produced
by stopping and starting a pump (Hinzen et al., 1972)

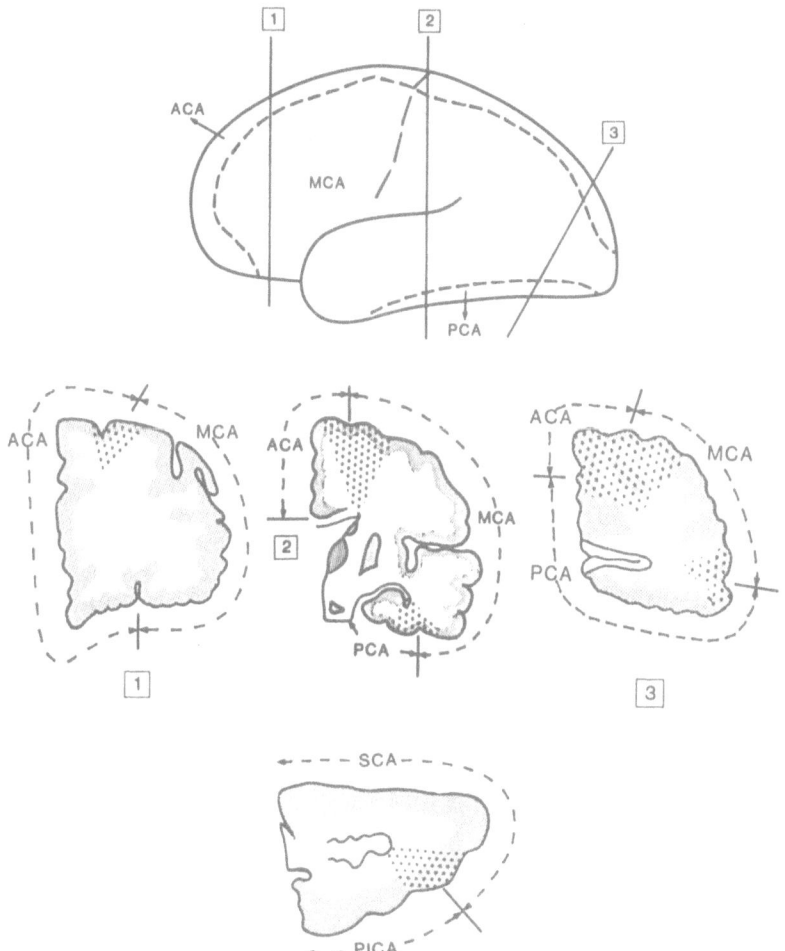

Fig. 5. Diagram to show arterial boundary zones in cerebral and
         cerebellar hemispheres. The right cerebral hemisphere is
         shown at three levels, viz. 1 = frontal, 2 = mid-temporal
         and 3 = occipital. Each boundary zone is stippled. ACA =
         anterior cerebral artery, MCA = middle cerebral artery,
         PCA = posterior cerebral artery, SCA = superior cerebellar
         artery and PICA = posterior inferior cerebellar artery.
         (Reproduced by kind permission of the Editor of the British
         Medical Journal from Graham, J.Clin.Path., 30,Suppl. (Roy.
         Coll.Path), 11:170-180.

     In a brief review Brierley (1980) considered that recent studies
in experimental animals fell into three main groups. In one group
the animals were paralyzed and mechanically ventilated and brain

ischaemia was produced by a combination of an inflated cuff to oc-
clude major neck arteries and drug-induced hypotension to eliminate
inflow through the collateral vessels (Nemoto et al., 1977). The
animals were maintained in an optimal physiological state by stan-
dardized intensive care with 24 hours coverage by trained personnel.
By these means Nemoto et al. (1977) concluded that the ischaemic
threshold of the brain in the rhesus monkey is about 15 minutes, a
figure which is similar to the 14-15 minute threshold determined by
Miller and Myers (1970). A somewhat similar approach has been used
in a second group of experiments that have employed a combination of
major arterial occlusion and drug-induced hypotension (Hossmann and
Sato, 1970; Hossmann and Zimmerman, 1974; Miller et al., 1980). In
the studies reported by Hossmann cerebral circulatory arrest for up
to 60 minutes has been followed by some recovery of neuronal function
as shown by the return of an abnormal EEG and a considerable restoration of brain energy metabolism. Such findings have been used to
conclude that the brain is able to tolerate a much longer period of
ischaemia than thought previously (Schneider, 1963). Hirsch et al.
(1975) however have failed to confirm the findings of Hossman and
Sato (1970) and attributed recovery after such protracted ischaemia
to the protective effects of anaesthesia and hypothermia. In a third
group of experiments cerebral circulatory arrest has been obtained by
raising the pressure of the CSF above that of the systolic blood
pressure. This method has been used in the rat (Brierley et al.,
1975) and rabbit (Marshall et al., 1975) with the production of
ischaemic cell change in the cerebral cortex and hippocampus after an
arrest of 10-15 minutes. The relevance of this particular model to
clinical medicine remains uncertain.

Oligaemic

    Global oligaemia implies some reduction in the overall flow of
blood through the brain. Because of autoregulation a moderate fall
in mean arterial blood pressure (about 60 mmHg) does not lead to a
reduction in CBF. Below the lower limit of autoregulation, however,
when vasodilatation is maximal, CBF will fall parallel to the perfusion pressure (see chapter by W. Fitch). Experimental studies in
the rhesus monkey have shown that if arterial oxygenation remains
normal, cerebral perfusion pressure must be reduced to 25 mmHg. for
at least 15 minutes before brain damage is produced (Brierley et al.,
1969; Meldrum and Brierley, 1969). In these animals hypoxic brain
damage was restricted to the arterial boundary zones of the cortex of
the cerebrum and also of the cerebellum. These experiments clearly
demonstrated that in the healthy spontaneously breathing primate
global oligaemia per se is unlikely to lead to brain damage if respiration does not fail.

    A comparable pattern of hypoxic brain damage was produced in a
very different physiological setting by Brierley et al. (1980).

Lightly anaesthetized and spontaneously breathing baboons inhaled an oxygen-nitrogen mixture producing a PaO_2 of 22-25 mmHg for about 20 minutes. Occlusion of one common carotid artery was without effect and when the other artery was occluded 15 minutes later, breathing was unaffected but eventually the EEG declined and became iso-electric. When carotid flow was restored and air breathing resumed after 10-15 minutes of the isoelectric state, the EEG returned at a very variable rate and was often abnormal. Microscopic examination of the brains showed hypoxic damage invariably along the boundary zones between the distribution of the anterior and middle cerebral arteries. It is concluded that in these animals maximal vasodila-tation had been produced during the initial hypoxaemia but flow through the carotid system only attained a critical level after occlusion of the second artery and then only in the boundary zone.

Further instances of the boundary zone pattern of hypoxic damage have been found after the intracarotid injection of air (Nicholson et al., 1970) and in both halothane and trimetaphan-induced hypotension in hypertensive baboons (Fitch et al., 1978; Graham et al., 1982). In these latter experiments CBF became pressure dependent below an arterial pressure of about 90 mmHg., i.e. at a higher level of arterial pressure than the lower limit of autoregulation (60 mmHg) in the normotensive baboon. These findings therefore indicated that there had been the expected shift to the right of the lower limit of autoregulation as a consequence of the structural changes that had taken place in the walls of the small vessels of the hypertensive animals.

Additional factors that may result in brain damage after a period of relatively moderate hypotension are some degree of hypox-aemia, some element of pre-existing desease, particularly atheroma of the extracranial and/or intracranial arteries and arteriosclerosis, and congenital variations of the circle of Willis. The frequency of these factors in addition to the reduction in CBF due to systemic hypotension is largely responsible for the observation that neuronal necrosis along the arterial boundary zones is the most common neuro-pathological outcome of hypoxia in all its forms.

CONCEPT OF THRESHOLDS ISCHAEMIA

The relationship between the blood supply and the capacity of a nerve cell to function and maintain its structural integrity remains of fundamental importance. Thus, according to the classical view (Schneider, 1963), if cardiac arrest is of abrupt onset and occurs in patients at normal body temperature, complete clinical recovery is unlikely if the period of arrest is more than 4-5 minutes. Both clinical and experimental experience, however, suggests that some recovery can be expected even if the period of circulatory arrest extends to 10-15 minutes. This has given rise to the hypothesis that certain nerve cells probably survive in a state of structural integrity but functional paralysis. From this has developed the concept of ischaemic thresholds (Astrup et al., 1977, 1979; Branston et al., 1977; Symon et al., 1977) according to which at certain low and decreasing levels of CBF the supply of oxygen becomes insufficient to support spontaneous and evoked electrical activity followed by failure of the NA^+-K^+ plump: it is only at very low levels of cerebral blood flow (about 10ml/100g/min) that nerve cells become irreversibly damaged (Astrup et al., 1981). More recent work, however, has shown that whilst the concept of ischaemic thresholds is valuable, the absolute levels of CBF at which the various derangements of neuronal function become manifest are likely to vary depending, amongst other things, upon the age and species of experimental animal, the particular model of hypoxia under study, temperature, whether the animals are conscious or anaesthetized, etc.

CONCLUSIONS

It will be evident from this brief review that ischaemic cell change is probably the cytopathological common denominator in all types of hypoxic brain damage. With the exception of circulatory arrest, however, there is no pattern of its distribution specific for each category of hypoxia. In the remaining categories, including oligaemic stagnant hypoxia, brain damage occurs principally along the arterial boundary zones. There is now ample evidence to show in the intact, healthy, spontaneously breathing animal tolerance to hypoxia is limited by the respiratory and circulatory systems and not by the intrinsic energy reserves of the brain itself.

It should be stressed that several types of hypoxia, each constituting a relatively mild stress, can in combination produce brain damage. Additional factors most probably responsible for the increased extent and frequency of brain damage in man include pre-existing cardiac disease which will impair the capacity to maintain a high level of blood flow through a cerebrovasular bed initially fully dilated by hypoxia, pre-existing disease in the arteries of the brain and neck, congenital variations of the circle of Willis, and any impairment of the normal reactivity of the smaller cerebral vessels.

Experiments in physiologically monitored spontaneously breathing animals have shown that hypoxia gives rise to an integrated series of responses in the respiratory, cardiovascular and nervous systems. Initially these serve to maintain brain function and respiration in particular. Ultimately these compensatory responses fail and under these circumstances brain damage is probably due to a failure of cerebral perfusion.

Acknowledgements

I am grateful to the Department of Medical Illustration, Southern General Hospital, for photographic assistance and to Mrs. J. Rubython for typing the manuscript.

REFERENCES

Adams, J. H., Brierley, J. B., Connor, R. C. R., and Treip, C. S., 1966, The effects of systemic hypotension upon the human brain. Clinical and neuropathological observations in 11 cases, Brain, 89:235-268.

Adams, J. H., Graham, D. I., Mills, E., and Sprunt, T. G., 1972, Fat embolism and cerebral infarction after use of methylmethacrylic cement, Brit.Med.J., 3:740-741.

Agardh, C -D., Kalimo, H., Olsson, Y., and Siesjö, B. K., 1981, Letter to editor, Acta Neuropathol.(Berl) 55:323-325.

Arsénio-Nunes, M. L., Hossmann, K. -A., Farkas-Bargeton, E., 1973, Ultrastructural and histochemical investigation of the cerebral cortex of cat during and after complete ischemia, Acta Neuropathol.(Berl) 26:329-344.

Astrup, J., Blennow, G., and Nilsson, B., 1979, Effects of reduced cerebral blood flow on EEG pattern, cerebral extracellular potassium and energy metabolism in the rat cortex during bicuculline-induced seizure, Brain Res., 177:115-126.

Astrup, J., Symon, L., Branston, N. M., and Lassen, N. A., 1977, Cortical evoked potential and extracellular K^+ and H^+ at critical levels of brain ischemia, Stroke, 8:51-57.

Branston, N. M., Strong, A. J., and Symon, L., 1977, Extracellular potassium activity, evoked potential and tissue blood flow, J.Neurol.Sci., 32:305-321.

Brierley, J. B., 1976, Cerebral hypoxia, in: "Greenfield's Neuropathology," 3rd edit. W. Blackwood and J. A. N. Corsellis, eds., pp.43-86, Arnold, London.

Brierley, J. B., 1980, Hypoxic brain damage, in: "Animal Models of Neurological Disease," F. C. Rose and P. O. Behan, eds., pp.338-346, Pitman Medical, Tunbridge Wells.

Brierley, J. B., Brown, A. W., Excell, B. J., and Meldrum, B. S., 1969, Brain damage in the Rhesus monkey resulting from profound hypotension. I. Its nature, distribution and general physiological correlates, Brain Res., 13:68-100.

Brierley, J. B., and Brown, A. W. (1981), Letter to the editor, Acta Neuropathol.(Berl), 55:319-322.

Brierley, J. B., Ljunggren, B., and Siesjö, B. K., 1975, Neuropathological alterations in rat brain after complete ischaemia due to raised intracranial pressure, in: "Intracranial Pressure II", N. Lundberg, U. Ponten and M. Brock, eds., pp.166-171, Springer, Berlin; Heidelberg, New York.

Brierley, J. B., and Miller, A. A., 1966, Fatal brain damage after
    dental anaesthesia. Its nature, aetiology and prevention,
    Lancet, ii:869–873.
Brierley, J. B., Prior, P. F., Calverley, J., Jackson, S. J., and
    Brown, A. W., 1980, The pathogenesis of ischaemic neuronal
    damage along the cerebral arterial boundary zones in Papio
    Anubis, Brain, 103:929–965.
Brown, A. W., 1977, Structural abnormalities in neurones, in:
    "Hypoxia and Ischaemia," B. C. Morson, ed., J.Clin.Path.,
    30:Suppl. (Roy.Coll.Path), 11:155–169.
Fitch, W., Jones, J. V., Graham, D. I., MacKenzie, E. T., and Harper,
    A. M., 1978, Effects of hypotension induced by halothane on
    the cerebral circulation in baboons with experimental reno-
    vascular hypertension, Brit.J.Anaesth., 50:119–125.
Garcia, J. H., Kalimo, H., Kamijyo, Y., and Trump, B. F., 1977, Cel-
    lular events during partial cerebral ischemia. I. Electron
    microscopy of feline cerebral cortex and middle cerebral
    artery occlusion, Virchows Arch.B.Cell Pathol., 25:191–206.
Graham, D. I., 1975, Ischaemic brain damage of cerebral perfusion
    failure type after treatment of severe hypertension, Brit.
    Med.J., 4:739.
Graham, D. I., 1977, Pathology of hypoxic brain damage in man, in:
    "Hypoxia and Ischaemia," B. C. Morson, ed., J.Clin.Path., 30:
    (Roy.Coll.Path.), 11:170–180.
Graham, D. I., Adams, J. H., and Doyle, D., 1978, Ischaemic brain
    damage in fatal non-missile head injuries, J.Neurol.Sci.,
    39:213–234.
Graham, D. I., McGeorge, A., Fitch, W., Jones, J. V., and MacKenzie,
    E. T., 1982, Rapidly induced hypotension in hypertensive
    baboons, Submitted to Clinical and Experimental Hypertension.
Hendrickx, H. H. L., Gisvold, S. E., Safar, P., and Swint, K., 1981,
    A new cardiac arrest rat model for brain resuscitation
    studies, J.Cerebral Blood Flow and Metab., 1:Suppl.1,
    S222–S223.
Hinzen, D. H., Muller, U., Sobotka, P., Lang, G. R., and Hirsch, H.,
    1972, Metabolism and function of dogs' brain recovering from
    long time ischemia, Amer.J.Physiol., 223:1158–1164.
Hirsch, H., Oberdorster, G., Zimmer, R., Benner, K. U., and Lang, R.,
    1975, The recovery of the electrocorticogram of normothermic
    canine brains after complete ischemia, Arch.f.Psychiat.u.
    Nervenkrank., 221:171–179.
Hossman, K. A., and Sato, K., 1970, Recovery of neuronal function
    after prolonged cerebral ischemia, Science, 168:375–376.
Hossman, K. A., and Zimmermann, V., 1974, Resuscitation of the monkey
    brain after 1 hour complete ischemia. I. Physiological and
    morphological observations, Brain Res., 81:59–74.
Jenkins, L. W., Povlishock, J. T., Lewelt, W., Miller, J. D., and
    Becker, D. P., 1979b, The role of postischemic recirculation
    in the development of ischemic neuronal injury following
    complete cerebral ischemia, Acta Neuropathol.(Berl),
    55:205–220.

Jenkins, L. W., Povlishock, J. T., Becker, D. P., Miller, J. D., and
    Sullivan, H. G., 1979a, Complete cerebral ischemia. An ultra-
    structural study, Acta Neuropathol.(Berl), 48:113-125.
Jennett, B., and Plum, F., 1972, Persistent vegetative state after
    brain damage: a syndrome in search of a name, Lancet,
    i:734-737.
Kalimo, H., Garcia, J. H., Kamijyo, Y., Tanaka, J., and Trump, F.,
    1977, The ultrastructure of "brain death". II. Electron micro-
    scopy of feline cortex after complete ischemia, Virchows
    Arch.Cell Pathol., 25:207-220.
Lin, S. -R., O'Connor, M. J., King, A., Harnish, P., and Fischer,
    H. W., 1979, Effect of dextran on cerebral function and blood
    flow after cardiac arrest. An experimental study on the dog,
    Stroke, 10:13-20.
Marshall, L. F., Graham, D. I., Durity, F., Lounsbury, R., Welsh, F.,
    and Langfitt, T. W., 1975, Experimental cerebral oligemia and
    ischemia produced by intracranial hypertension. Part 2. Brain
    morphology, J.Neurosurg., 43:318-322.
Meldrum, B. S., and Brierley, J. B., 1969, Brain damage in the Rhesus
    monkey resulting from profound arterial hypotension. II.
    Changes in the spontaneous and evoked electrical activity of
    the neocortex, Brain Res., 13:101-118.
Miller, C. L., Lampard, D. G., Alexander, K., and Brown, W. A., 1980,
    Local cerebral blood flow following transient cerebral isch-
    emia. I. Onset of impaired reperfusion within the first hour
    following global ischemia, Stoke, 11:534-541.
Miller, J. R., and Myers, R. E., 1970, Neurological effects of
    systemic circulatory arrest in the monkey, Neurology
    (Minneap), 20:715-724.
Nemoto, E. M., Bleyaert, A. L., Stezoski, S. W., Moossy, J., Rao,
    G. R., and Safar, P., 1977, Global brain ischemia: a repro-
    ducible monkey model, Stroke, 8:558-564.
Nicholson, A. N., Freeland, S. A., and Brierley, J. B., 1970,
    A behavioural and neuropathological study of the sequelae of
    profound hypoxia, Brain Res., 22:327-345.
Patterson, R. S., McSherry, C. K., and Schwartz, M. S., 1968, Hyper-
    baric oxygen, hypothermia and cerebral ischaemia in the dog,
    J.Surg.Res., 8:279-285.
Plum, F., 1973, The clinical problem: how much anoxia-ischemia
    damages the brain? Arch.Neurol., 29:359-360.
Romanoul, F. C. A., and Abramowicz, A., 1964, Changes in brain and
    pial vessels in arterial border zones, Arch.Neurol., 11:40-65.
Schneider, M., 1963, Critical blood pressure in the cerebral
    circulation, in: "Selective Vulnerability of the Brain in
    Hypoxaemia," J. P. Schade and W. M. McMenemy, eds., pp.7-20,
    Blackwell, Oxford.
Symon, L., Branston, N. M., Strong, A. J., and Hope, T. D., 1977, The
    concepts of thresholds of ischaemia in relation to brain
    structure and function, J.Clin.Path., 30:Suppl. (Roy.Coll.
    Path.), 11:149-154.

STRUCTURAL CHANGES IN THE BRAIN DURING THE

CRITICAL REDUCTION OF BLOOD FLOW OR OXYGEN TENSION

H. Kalimo

Department of Pathology
University of Turku
SF-20520 Turku 52, Finland

Experimental studies on cerebral ischemia during the past ten years have demonstrated that even relatively long periods of complete ischemia may allow a considerable recovery of the cerebral energy state (Hossmann and Kleihues 1973; Nordström et al., 1978), mitochondrial respiratory function (e.g. Schutz et al., 1973; Ginsberg et al., 1977; Rehncrona et al., 1979), neurolphysiological parameters (Hossmann and Kleihues 1973; Rehncrona et al., 1980, 1981) and neurological function (Miller and Myers 1970; Safar et al., 1976). In contrast similar or even shorter insults of incomplete ischemia (e.g. Salford et al., 1973; Hossmann and Kleihues 1973; Nordström et al., 1978; Rehncrona et al., 1979) have been demonstrated to cause more severe brain damage.

Accordingly most structural studies have failed to disclose extensive neuronal damage after complete ischemia of 15-30 min or even up to 60 min duration (Arsenio-Nunes et al., 1973; Garcia et al., 1975; Kalimo et al., 1977, 1979; Jenkins et al. 1979), whereas apparently more severe structural damage has been encountered following similar periods of incomplete ischemia (e.g. Brown and Brierley 1972; Garcia et al., 1975, 1977). Thus paradoxically, continued yet insufficient blood supply to the brain seems to be more detrimental than a complete cut-off of all cerebral circulation, which implies that other factors besides the lack of oxygen contribute to the development of the ischemic tissue damage. These results also imply that certain optimal, still undefined conditions allow the brain to withstand surprisingly long periods of critically reduced blood flow or oxygen tension. Furthermore the structural changes caused by these adverse conditions seem to vary depending on the mode of the ischemic insult as well as the presence of recirculation.

CHARACTER OF THE STRUCTURAL CHANGES

The classic neuronal "ischemic cell change", which was originally described by Spielmeyer (1922) and later illustrated in greater detail (e.g. by Brown and Brierley 1966, 1972; Arsenio-Nunes et al., 1973; Garcia et al., 1975, 1977; and Jenkins et al., 1981), is characterized by initial microvacuolation due to mitochondrial ballooning followed by severe condensation of the neuronal cyto- and karyoplasm and swelling of the perineuronal as well as perivascular astrocytic processes. Finally homogenization and disappearance of the injured neurons occurs. This type of injury has been suggested to result from incomplete and/or transient ischemia (Garcia et al., 1975, 1977). Complete ischemia without recirculation gives less dramatic structural changes (Garcia et al., 1975; Kalimo et al., 1977, 1979; Jenkins et al., 1979): the nuclear chromatin becomes clumped and the cell sap increasingly electron lucent, mitochondria are slightly to moderately swollen as are often the cisternae of the endoplasmic reticulum, whereas the astrocytic swelling is less prominent (cf. Figures 1b, 1c and 2). Whether this type of change could transform into the classic vacuolated and condensed type of ischemic nerve cell injury is still an open question.

ROLE OF TISSUE LACTIC ACIDOSIS

To further elucidate which factors are crucial for rendering the ischemic nerve cell injury irreversible and to clarify which structural changes are indicative of irreversible damage, we examined the role of the lactic acidosis which develops in the brain tissue during the ischemic insult. As discussed by Rehncrona in this symposium, excessive brain lactic acidosis has a definite detrimental effect on the post-ischemic recovery of the cerebral energy state and neurophysiological parameters (see also Myers 1979; Rehncrona et al., 1981). In the same model of severe incomplete ischemia (induced in rats by bilateral clamping of carotid arteries and lowering of the mean arterial blood pressure to 50 mmHg for 30 min followed by recirculation for 0, 5 or 90 minutes; for details see Rehncrona et al., 1981) we also examined the light (LM) and electron microscopic (EM) changes. The degree of tissue lactic acidosis was varied by giving one group an infusion of glucose 15 min prior to the ischemia, whereas the other group was given saline. In the former, high lactic acidosis group the tissue lactate during the ischemia rose to ca. 35 μmol $\cdot$g^{-1}, whereas in the latter, low lactic acidosis group it remained at about 15 μmol $\cdot$g^{-1}.

In the low lactic acidosis group the structural changes in the cerebral cortex immediately after 30 min of severe imcomplete ischemia had a homogeneous distribution and - considering the duration of the ischemia - were surprisingly discrete. By LM (Figure 1b) the nuclear chromatin of neurons appeared slightly coarser than in the controls but it remained fairly evenly distributed. In astrocytes and oligodendrocytes the chromatin was somewhat clumped. The structure in general appeared slightly "blurred". After 5 min of recirculation the changes were about the same or even milder. Remarkably, the condensed, vacuolated type of ischemically injured neurons were very rarely present. Only around some larger penetrating arteries, where some edematous vacuolization was also seen, a few such injured neurons were encountered. Following 90 min of recirculation the cerebral cortex in the low lactic acidosis group appeared essentially indistinguishable from the controls (Figure 1c). Edematous vacuolization had disappeared, but very few (less than 0.1% of all neurons) condensed neurons remained, some being even fragmented suggesting irreversible damage.

The mildness of the ischemic injury in the low lactic acidosis group was confirmed by electron microscopy (Figure 2). The nuclear chromatin in the neurons was slightly coarser than in the controls. Cytoplasmic organelles also withstood the insult remarkably well. The neuronal mitochondria showed mild to moderate swelling after 0 or 5 min of recirculation, but after 90 min they appeared nearly normal. The only change which became accentuated with longer duration of the recirculation was the dispersion and disintegration of free ribosomes as well as their detachment from the endoplasmic reticulum. Such a change conforms well to the biochemical results showing post-ischemic impairment of protein synthesis (Cooper et al., 1977). Furthermore it could structurally reflect an injury that might be responsible for the "maturation" of the ischemic nerve cell injury during the recirculation period as described by Klatzo (1979).

In the high lactic acidosis group the structural changes were distinctly more extensive (Figure 1d and 3). Both by LM and EM after 0 or 5 min of recirculation severe clumping of nuclear chromatin was verified in all cells. Similarly the cell sap appeared watery with fluffy material around the clustered organelles. These changes became even more pronounced after 90 min of recirculation, but since adequate perfusion of the fixative was no longer possible in this group, artefactual changes must also have contributed to the end result. Remarkably, after 0 and 5 min of recirculation the structural changes were again homogeneous throughout the cortex and neither was there any significant number of the condensed, vacuolated type of injured neurons.

Since the only significant difference between the above described two groups is the degree of lactic acidosis, our structural results — in concordance with the biochemical and neurophysiological data (Rehncrona in this symposium and Rehncrona et al., 1981) — demonstrated that high tissue lactate concentration during ischemia has a definite detrimental effect. The exact mechanism of this adverse effect is not known, but the marked reduction of the intracellular pH is obviously one important factor. The very low pH in

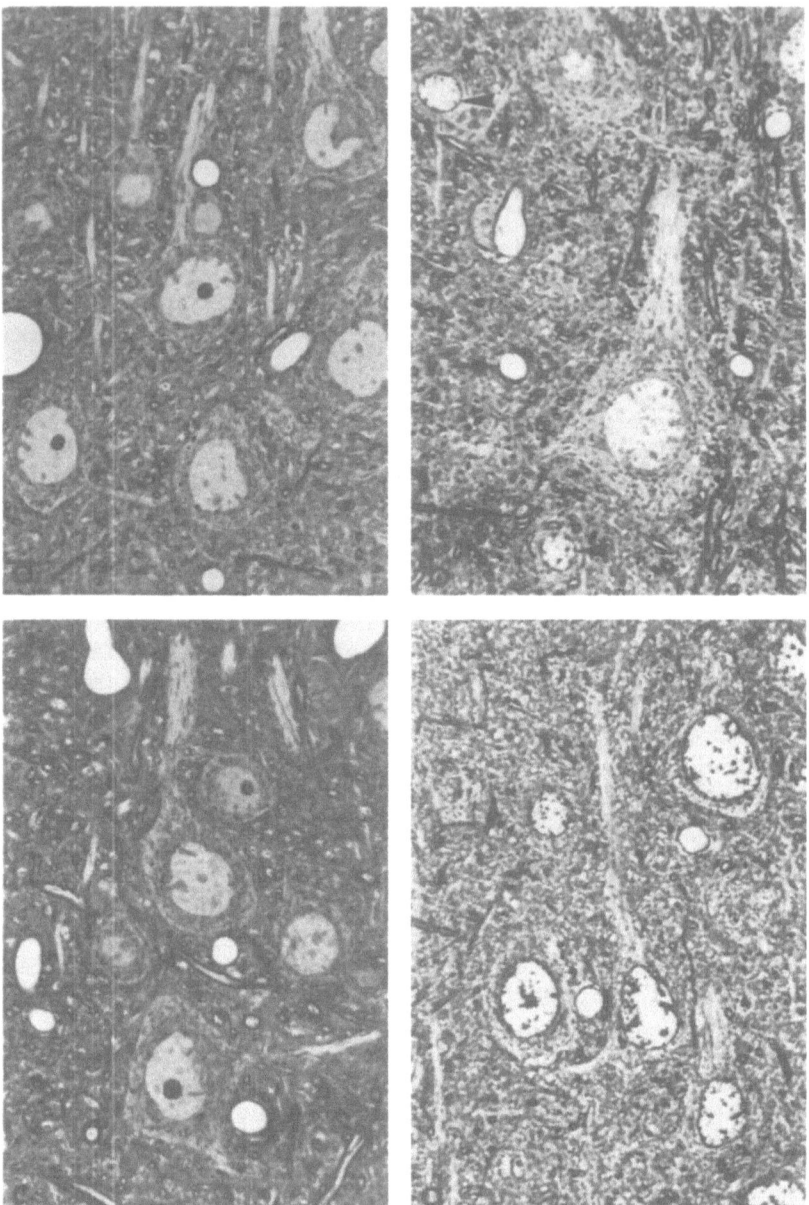

Fig. 1.   a) Light micrograph from cortical layer 5 of a control
          animal. 740 x.   b) Cortical layer 5 from a rat of the low
          lactic acidosis group exposed to 30 min of severe incomplete
          ischemia followed by 5 min of recirculation. Only minor
          changes are seen: chromatin is slightly coarse in neurons
          and clumped in astrocytes (arrowheads). The structure in
          general is somewhat "blurred". Capillaries are patent

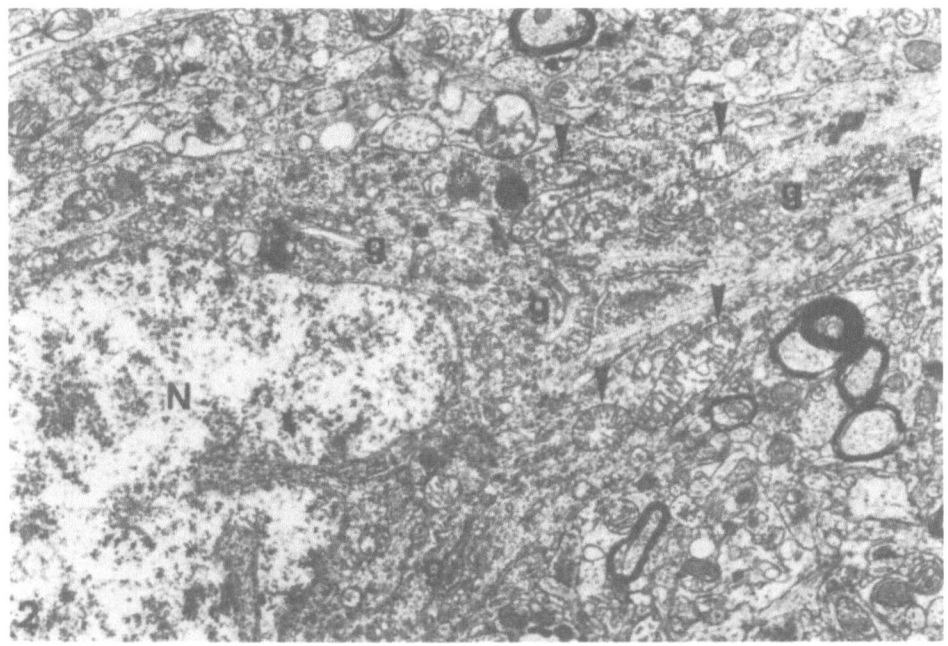

Fig. 2.   In the low lactic acidosis group also the EM changes are
          fairly discrete: nuclear chromatin (N) is coarse but rela-
          tively evenly distributed and mitochondria (arrowheads) show
          mild to moderate swelling, which is not severe enough to
          cause microvacuolization in LM. The rest of the organelles
          appear fairly intact (g = golgi apparatus). 8100 x.

the high lactic acidosis group (pH < 6.0) is most probably responsible for the severe clumping (denaturation?) of the nuclear chromatin. This view is corroborated by the studies on severe hypoglycemia (Agardh et al., 1980; Kalmio et al., 1980), in which an energy
failure also occurs, but the intracellular pH shifts instead towards
more alkaline values (Pelligrino et al., 1981), and thus neither the
nuclear chromatin nor the cell sap becomes clumped (Figure 4) as it
does in most anoxic ischemic conditions.

(arrows). 810 x. c) The same experimental group as in
Figures 1b after recirculation for 90 min. In LM the structure appears indistinguishable from the control. 740 x.
d) In the high lactic acidosis group with recirculation for
5 min the nuclear chromatin is severely clumped and cellular
details are less distinct, but no condensation or vacuolization of neurons is apparent. 740 x.

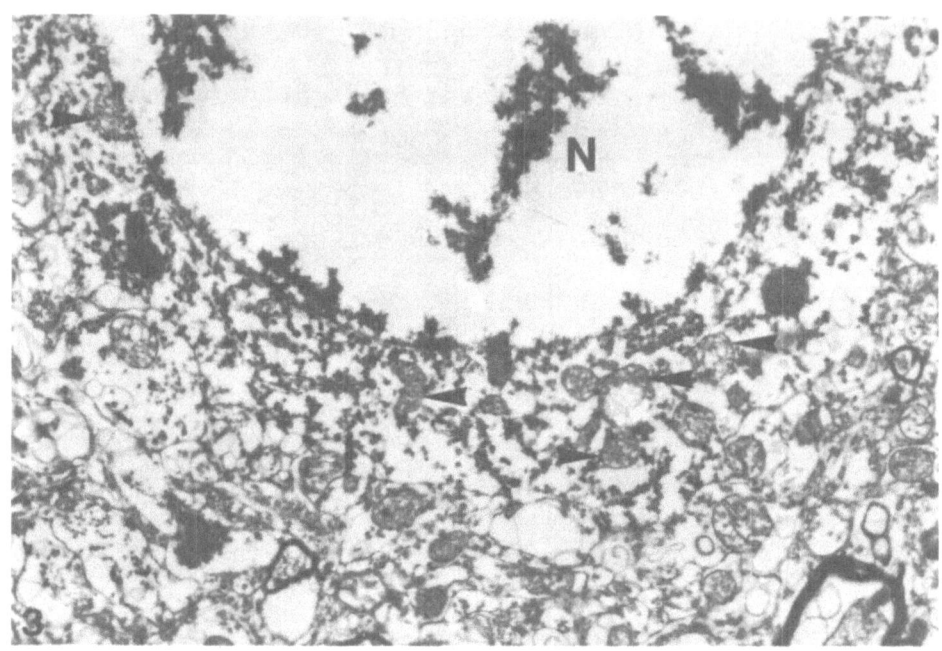

Fig. 3.   In the high lactic acidosis group the EM changes are
          prominent: nuclear chromatin (N) is severely clumped,
          the cytoplasm appears watery with fluffy material around
          the clustered organelles. Mitochondria (arrowheads) are
          slightly swollen. 9 100 x.

SIGNIFICANCE OF THE STRUCTURAL CHANGES OF ISCHEMIA

     It should be pointed out that in our study the recirculation
started well in both the low and high lactic acidosis groups, as also
indirectly evidenced by the patency of the capillaries in the microscopic preparations. Thus the "no-reflow phenomenon" cannot explain
the more severe damage in the high lactic acidosis group, in which
only later did the recirculation become progressively impaired. This
suggests that in this group the cells incurred an irreversible injury
during the ischemia, which doomed them to succumb. Additional damage
may occur during the recirculation period. In any case, the biochemical and nuerophysiological data (Rehncrona et al., 1981) imply
that the structural changes in the high lactic acidosis group most
likely represent irreversible tissue damage. On the other hand, the
marked recovery in the low lactic acidosis group suggests that the
injury is still reversible, at least in the short run. Assessment of
late effects such as the maturation phenemenon (Klatzo 1979) would
require considerably longer recirculation times.

     The paucity of the classic vacuolated, condensed injured neurons
(previously considered the hallmark of ischemic nerve cell injury) in

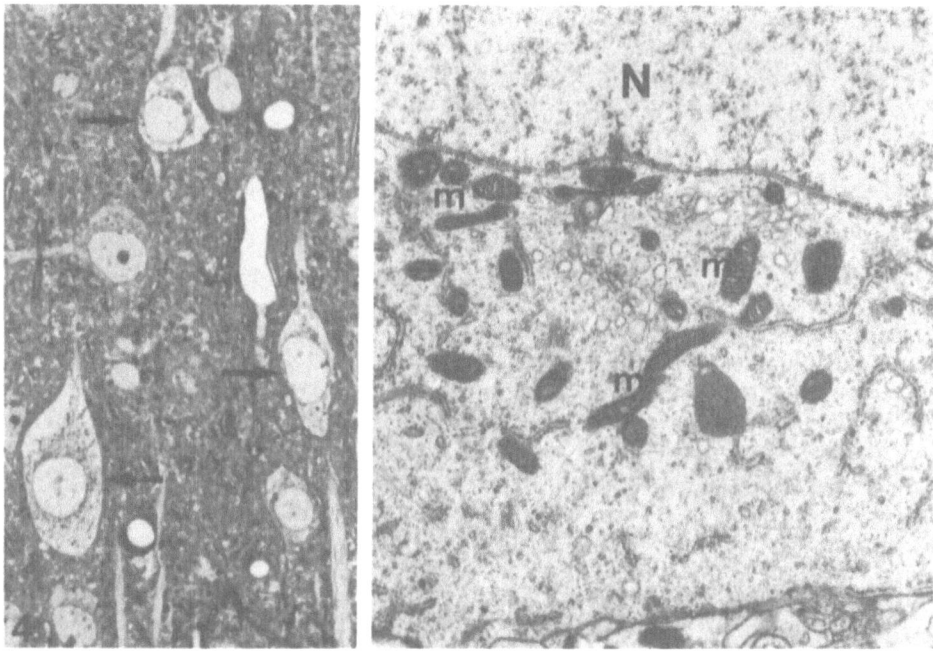

Fig. 4. In severe hypoglycemia (60 min with isoelectric EEG), which
         causes an energy failure but no intracellular acidosis, the
         clumping of nuclear chromatin or cytoplasm does not occur in
         the type 2 injured neurons (arrows). (N = nucleus, m = mito-
         chondrion). LM: epon + toluidine blue 700 x, EM: 10 350 x.

our model corroborates the view that there is more than one type of
ischemic nerve cell change. The reason why the evidently irreversibly injured neurons in the high lactic acidosis failed to
undergo vacuolization and condensation remains to be clarifed. A
possible explanation could be such as described in more detail by
Siesjö (1981). Condensation of neurons occurs only when ions leaking
from neurons stricken by energy failure are taken up by astrocytes
through an active, ATP-dependent mechanism. This shift of osmotic
equivalents accompanied by water (extra water coming from the residual or restored circulation?) results in active astrocytic swelling
and simultaneous neuronal condensation. This sequence requires
survival of astrocytes, which may be possible even when neurons fail,
since astrocytes can withstand lower oxygen tension than neurons and
besides they lie closer to the capillaries. In our high lactic
acidosis group the tissue damage may well have been severe enough to
knock out also most astrocytes and therefore so few condensed, vacuolated neurons were produced. Thus the condensed, vacuolated neurons,
are likely to appear in less severe or repeated ischemic insults.

    In conclusion, the brain might under optimal conditions tolerate
markedly more severe anoxia-ischemia than generally thought. A high

degree of tissue lactic acidosis during cerebral ischemia is one factor which impairs post-ischemic recovery and thus excessive blood glucose concentrations should be avoided when the cerebral blood flow or oxygen tension are critically reduced.

REFERENCES

Agardh, C. D., Kalimo, H., Olsson, Y., and Siesjö, B. K., 1980, Hypo-glycemic brain injury. I. Metabolic and light microscopic findings in rat cerebral cortex during profound insulin-induced hypoglycemia and in recovery period following glucose administration, Acta Neuropathol., 50:31-41.

Arsenio-Nunes, M. L., Hossmann, K. A., and Farkas-Bargeton, E., 1973, Ultrastructural and histochemical investigation of the cere-bral cortex of cat during and after complete ischemia, Acta Neuropathol., 26:329-344.

Brown, A. W., and Brierley, J. B., 1966, Evidence for early anoxic-ischaemic cell damage in the rat brain, Experientia, 22:546-547.

Brown, A. W., and Brierley, J. B., 1972, Anoxic-ischemic cell change in rat brain. Light microscopic and fine-structural observ-ations, J.Neurol.Sci., 16:59-84.

Cooper, H. K., Zalewska, T., Kawakami, S., Hossman, K. A., and Kleihues, P., 1977, The effect of ischemia and recirculation on protein synthesis in the rat brain, J.Neurochem., 28:929-934.

Garcia, J. H., Kamijyo, Y., Kalimo, H., Tanaka, J., Viloria, J. E., and Trump, B. F., 1975, Cerebral ischemia: The early struc-tural changes and correlation of these with known metabolic and dynamic abnormalities, in: "Cerebral Vascular Diseases," J. P. Whisnant, B. Sandok, ed., Grune and Stratton, pp.313-323, New York.

Garcia, J. H., Kalimo, H., Kamijyo, Y., and Trump, B. F., 1977, Cel-lular events during partial cerebral ischemia. I. Electron microscopy of feline cerebral cortex after middle-cerebral-artery occlusion, Virchows Arch.Cell.Pathol., 25:191-206.

Ginsberg, M. D., Mela, L., Wrobel-Kuhl, K., and Reivich, M., 1977, Mitochondrial metabolism following bilateral cerebral ischemia in the gerbil, Ann Neurol., 1:519-527.

Hossmann, K. A., and Kleihues, P., 1973, Reversibility of ischemic brain damage, Arch.Neurol., 29:375-382.

Jenkins, L. W., Povlishock, J. T., Becker, D. P., Miller, J. D., and Sullivan, H. G., 1979, Complete cerebral ischemia. An ultra-structural study, Acta Neuropathol., 48:113-125.

Jenkins, L. W., Povlishock, J. T., Lewelt, W., Miller, J. D., and Becker, D. P., 1981, The role of post-ischemic recirculation in the development of ischemic neuronal injury following complete cerebral ischemia, Acta Neuropathol., 55:205-220.

Kalimo, H., Garcia, J. H., Kamijyo, Y., Tanaka, J., and Trump, F.,

1977, The ultrastructure of "brain death." II. Electron microscopy of feline cortex after complete ischemia, Virchows
Arch.Cell.Pathol., 25:207-220.

Kalimo, H., Paljärvi, L., and Vapalahti, M., 1979, The early ultra-
structural alterations in the rabbit cerebral and cerebellar
cortex after compression ischaemia, Neuropathol.Appl.
Neurobiol., 5:211-223.

Kalimo, H., Rehncrona, S., Söderfeldt, B., Olsson, Y., and Siesjö,
B. K., 1981, Brain lactic acidosis and ischemic cell damage:
2. Histopathology, J.Cereb.Blood Flow Metab., 1:313-327.

Klatzo, I., 1979, Cerebral edema and ischemia, in: "Recent Advances
in Neuropathology," Vol.1, W. T. Smith, J. B. Cavanagh, ed.,
Churchill Livingstone, pp.27-40, Edinburgh.

Miller, J. R., and Myers, R. E., 1970, Neurological effects of
systemic circulatory arrest in the monkey, Neurology,
20:715-724.

Myers, R. E., 1979, A unitary theory of causation of anoxic and
hypoxic brain pathology, in: "Advances in Neurology, Vol.26:
Cerebral Hypoxia and its Consequences," S. Fahn, J. N. Davis,
L. P. Rowland, Raven Press, pp.195-213, New York.

Nordström, C. H., Rehncrona, S., and Siesjö, B. K., 1978, Restitution
of cerebral energy state, as well as of glycolytic metabolites, citric acid cycle intermediates and associated amino
acids after 30 min of complete ischemia in rats anesthetized
with nitrous oxide or phenobarbital, J.Neurochem., 30:479-486.

Pelligrino, D., Almquist, L. O., and Siesjö, B. K., 1981, Effects of
insulin-induced hypoglycemia on intracellular pH and impedance
in the cerebral cortex of the rat, Brain Research,
221:129-147.

Rehncrona, S., Mela, L., and Siesjö, B. K., 1979, Recovery of brain
mitochondrial function in the rat after complete and incomplete cerebral ischemia, Stroke, 10:437-446.

Rehncrona, S., Folbergrovà, J., Smith, N. S., and Siesjö, B. K.,
1980, Influence of complete and pronounced incomplete cerebral
ischemia and subsequent recirculation on cortical concentrations of oxidized and reduced glutathione in the rat,
J.Neurochem., 34:477-486.

Rehncrona, S., Rosèn, I., and Siesjö, B. K., 1981, Brain lactic
acidosis and ischemic cell damage: 1. Biochemistry and neurophysiology, J.Cereb.Blood Flow Metab., 1:297-311.

Safar, P., Stezoki, W., and Nemoto, E. M., 1976, Amelioration of
brain damage after 12 minutes cardiac arrest in dogs, Archives
of Neurology, 33:91-95.

Salford, L. G., Plum, F., and Siesjö, B. K., 1973, Graded hypoxia-
oligemia in rat brain. I. Biochemical alterations and their
implications, Arch.Neurol., 29:227-233.

Schutz, H., Silverstein, P. R., Vapalahti, M., Bruce, D. A., Mela,
L., and Langfitt, T. W., 1973, Brain mitochondrial function
after ischemia and hypoxia. I. Ischemia induced by increased
intracranial pressure, Arch.Neurol., 29:408-416.

Siesjö, B. K., 1981, Cell damage in the brain: A speculative
    synthesis, J.Cereb.Blood Flow Metabol., 1:155-185.
Spielmeyer, W., 1922, "Histopathologie des Nervensystems," Springer-
    Verlag, Berlin.

THE SIGNIFICANCE OF LOW O_2-TENSIONS IN THE BRAIN
CORTEX FOR OCCURRENCE OF METABOLIC ALTERATIONS
UNDER CRITICAL FLOW CONDITIONS

J. Grote, K. Zimmer, R.Schubert*

Department of Physiology, University of Bonn
5300 Bonn, FRG and Department of Neurosurgery*
University of Mainz, 6500 Mainz, FRG

A reduction in the O_2 supply to the brain cortex leads to O_2
deficiency and curtailment of neuronal metabolism and function as
soon as a minimal cellular O_2 tension of 0.1 - 1 mmHG (13 - 133 Pa)
can no longer be maintained (Chance et al., 1964; Grote 1967). The
hypoxia-induced metabolic alterations are characterized by decreased
tissue levels of the energy-rich phosphate compounds PCr and ATP. In
addition, elevated concentrations of lactate, pyruvate and NADH and
an increase in the lactate/pyruvate ratio and in the $NADH/NAD^+$ ratio
are to be expected (Duffy et al., 1972; Granholm and Siesjö 1969;
Granholm et al., 1969; Granholm and Siesjö 1971; Grote 1978; Grote
and Schubert 1982; Norberg and Siesjö 1975; Norberg et al., 1975;
Opitz and Schneider 1950; Schmahl et al., 1966).

Among the various pathophysiological conditions which induce
insufficient brain tissue oxygenation, arterial hypoxia and arterial
hypocapnia are of great importance (Granholm and Siesjö 1969;
Granholm et al., 1969; Granholm and Siesjö 1971; Grote et al., 1981;
Grote and Schubert 1982; Norberg and Siesjö 1975; Norberg et al.,
1975; Opitz and Schneider 1950). In order to study the threshold for
cortical O_2 supply at decreased arterial O_2 tension or arterial CO_2
tension, regional cerebral blood flow and tissue PO_2 measurements as
well as tissue metabolite assays were performed in the brain cortex
of cats.

METHODS

In both experimental series the animals were lightly anaesthetized with sodium pentobarbital (Nembutal, 25 mg/kg i.v.), completely
immobilized (Imbretil, 1.6 - 2.0 mg initially, 0.2 - 0.3 mg every

181

30 min) and artificially ventilated. In the first group of experiments normocapnic hypoxia conditions were established by adjusting
the O_2 fraction of the respiratory gas mixture. In the second group
tidal volume and ventilation frequency were increased to induce
normoxic hypocapnia. During the experiments endtidal CO_2 concentration was continuously recorded, while arterial PO_2 and pH were
intermittently determined. For blood sampling and blood pressure
measurements one femoral artery and the superior sagittal sinus were
catheterized. After bilateral craniotomy and opening of the dura
over the parietal cortex of both hemispheres, rCBF and tissue PO_2
were measured in the left and right suprasylvian gyri employing the
Kr^{85} clearance technique and multiwire surface PO_2 micro electrodes,
respectively (Grote et al., 1981; Hutten and Brock 1969; Kessler and
Grunewald 1978; Lübbers 1973; Lübbers et al., 1969; Zierler 1965).

     At the end of the experiments frozen tissue samples were taken
from the cortical areas under investigation to assay enzymatically
the concentrations of different metabolites in the cortical grey
matter (Grote et al., 1981). Additionally, tissue water content of
the grey and the subcortical white matter was determined by drying
the samples to constant weight for ruling out the occurence of brain
edema. Control values for the metabolite concentrations in the brain
cortex of cats during arterial normoxia and normocapnia were derived
from experiments performed under comparable conditions.

RESULTS AND DISCUSSION

     In the first series of experiments on 15 cats the arterial PO_2
was stepwise lowered from normal values to ca. 50 mmHg (6.7 kPa) and
to ca. 30 mmHg (4.0 kPa), maintaining both hypoxia levels for about
30 to 45 minutes. The arterial CO_2 tension as well as the mean
arterial blood pressure remained normal during the entire experiment,
Moderate arterial hypoxia produced the typical increase of regional
cortical blood flow (see Table 1) which, according to the metabolic
hypothesis of cerebral blood flow regulation (Betz 1972; Kuschinsky
and Wahl 1978), may be explained as the consequence of an imbalance
between O_2 supply and O_2 demand of the brain tissue. Under conditions of pronounced hypoxia, regional cortical blood flow was
further enhanced in all experiments reaching a mean value of 157.8
ml $\cdot$ $100g^{-1}$ $\cdot$ min^{-1}, which was approximately 50% above the initial
flow rate. In hypoxia experiments on cats with intact dura com-
parable blood flow reactions were found in the brain cortex, however, the mean blood flow rates at the different PaO_2 levels were
significantly lower (Grote and Schubert 1982).

     The tissue PO_2 values simultaneously measured are summarized in
PO_2 histograms. As can be seen in Figure 1 the mean tissue PO_2
distribution determined in the superficial cell layers of the brain
cortex during arterial normoxia, agrees with values derived from
needle electrode measurements in deeper cortical structures under

Table 1. Effects of Arterial Hypoxia and Arterial Hypocapnia on Regional Cortical Blood Flow. Mean Values ± SE are given.

	Normoxia	Moderate hypoxia	Severe hypoxia
n	15	14	8
PaO_2 (mmHg)	96.3 ± 3.2	51.8 ± 1.6	31.0 ± 2.0
$PaCO_2$ (mmHg)	28.5 ± 0.5	28.0 ± 0.5	27.0 ± 1.0
pHa	7.482 ± 0.011	7.471 ± 0.019	7.436 ± 0.030
rCBF ($ml \cdot 100g^{-1} \cdot min^{-1}$)	111.0 ± 8.9	125.9 ± 13.7	157.8 ± 14.7

	Normocapnia	Moderate hypocapnia	Severe hypocapnia
N	12	12	12
PaO_2 (mmHg)	100.0 ± 4.7	111.9 ± 6.0	111.6 ± 4.4
$PaCO_2$ (mmHg)	29.5 ± 0.5	18.8 ± 0.4	12.1 ± 0.3
pHa	7.411 ± 0.013	7.509 ± 0.032	7.619 ± 0.031
rCBF ($ml \cdot 100g^{-1} \cdot min^{-1}$)	129.2 ± 4.0	103.1 ± 3.4	97.6 ± 5.1

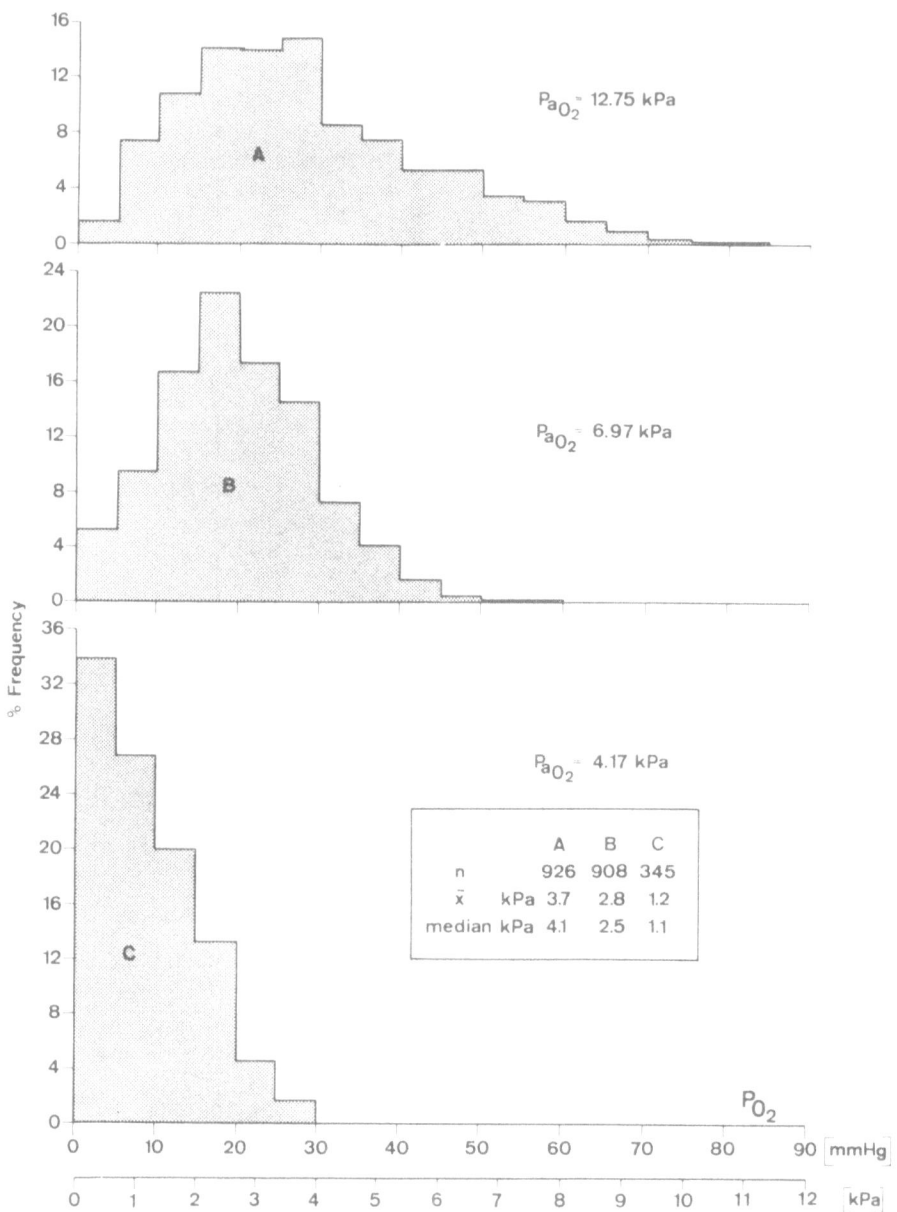

Fig. 1. PO$_2$ histograms of the brain cortex of cats determined during
arterial normoxia and arterial hypoxia (PaO$_2$ = 52 mmHg and
31 mmHg respectively).

comparable conditions (Leniger-Follert et al., 1975; Lübbers 1973).
The cortical oxygen tensions were found between very low values near
0 mmHg and arterial oxygen tension with a mean value of 27.7 mmHg

(3.7 kPa). After decreasing the arterial oxygen tension to ca.
50 mmHg (6.7 kPa) a pronounced shift of the tissue PO$_2$ frequency
distribution to low oxygen tensions could be observed. The tissue
oxygen tension values between 0 and 2.5 mmHg (0 - 333 Pa) significantly increased, indicating the presence of tissue hypoxia with
anoxia in single cells. Since at the same time elevated regional
cortical blood flow rates were found, the results suggest that a more
pronounced brain cortex hypoxia was present before cerebral vasodilation induced the rCBF increase. Moreover, the very low tissue
oxygen tensions still present at high flow rates may induce the
maintenance of the hyperemia. The lowering of arterial oxygen tension to ca. 30 mmHg resulted in severe cortical hypoxia with a mean
tissue PO$_2$ value of 9 mmHg (1.2 kPA).

The results of the metabolite assays which are given in Table 2
confirm the above assumptions. During moderate arterial hypoxia the
tissue concentrations of lactate and pyruvate as well as the lactate/
pyruvate ratio were elevated indicating the acceleration of glycolysis. At the same time the phosphocreatine concentration was significantly decreased. The ATP concentration was slightly below the
normal level, while the tissue concentrations of ADP and AMP were
above the values measured at arterial normoxia. The increase in
glycolysis may be due to the observed changes in the tissue concentrations of phosphocreatine and ADP which induce an activation of the
phosphofructokinase, the major regulatory enzyme of the glycolytic
pathway (Norberg and Siesjö 1975; Norberg et al., 1975). During
pronounced arterial hypoxia all changes of the tissue metabolite
concentrations were enhanced, demonstrating that in spite of the
elevated regional cortical blood flow rates the reduction of mean
arterial oxygen tensions to 31 mmHg (4.1 kPa) produced a severe
imbalance between O$_2$ supply and O$_2$ demand in the brain cortex.

In the second experimental group 12 cats were hyperventilated to
reduce the arterial CO$_2$ tension to ca. 20 mmHg (2.7 kPa) and ca.
12 mmHg (1.6 kPa). Arterial hypocapnia produced the typical increase
of cerebrovascular resistance and a subsequent decrease of mean
regional cortical blood flow. However, at arterial CO$_2$ tensions of
ca. 12 mmHg an inhomogeneous blood flow pattern was observed. The
simultaneously performed blood flow measurements in the two corresponding regions of the right and left hemisphere showed further
decreased as well as increased flow rates.

The tissue PO$_2$ frequency histograms determined for normocapnia
and hypocapnia conditions are given in Figure 2. During arterial
normocapnia the oxygen measurements on the brain cortex resulted in
all cases in typical PO$_2$ histograms, agreeing with those performed
under similar conditions in the first group of experiments. Under
arterial hypocapnia, due to the blood flow reduction as well as to
the displacement of the blood O$_2$ dissociation curve, the oxygen
transfer from blood to tissue was decreased resulting in a shift of

Table 2. The Effect of Moderate (PaO_2 = 50 mmHg = 6.7 kPa) and Severe Arterial Hypoxia (PaO_2 = 30 mmHg = 4.0 kPa) as well as of Severe Arterial Hypocapnia ($PaCO_2$ = 12.0 mmHg = 1.6 kPa) on Tissue Metabolites in the Brain Cortex of Cats. Metabolite Concentrations are given as $\mu mol \cdot g^{-1}$ Wet Weight. Mean Values ± SE are given.

	Normoxia-normocapnia	Moderate hypoxia	Severe hypoxia	Severe hypocapnia
La	1.244 ± 0.141	10.166 ± 2.727	23.737 ± 3.674	5.915 ± 1.094
Py	0.096 ± 0.020	0.096 ± 0.020	0.247 ± 0.044	0.220 ± 0.027
PCr	4.59 ± 0.20	2.24 ± 0.52	1.07 ± 0.25	3.38 ± 0.25
ATP	2.53 ± 0.15	2.26 ± 0.08	1.96 ± 0.22	2.58 ± 0.15
ADP	0.33 ± 0.03	0.53 ± 0.06	0.75 ± 0.11	0.54 ± 0.08
AMP	0.04 ± 0.01	0.18 ± 0.03	0.15 ± 0.03	0.07 ± 0.02
n	10	5	13	9

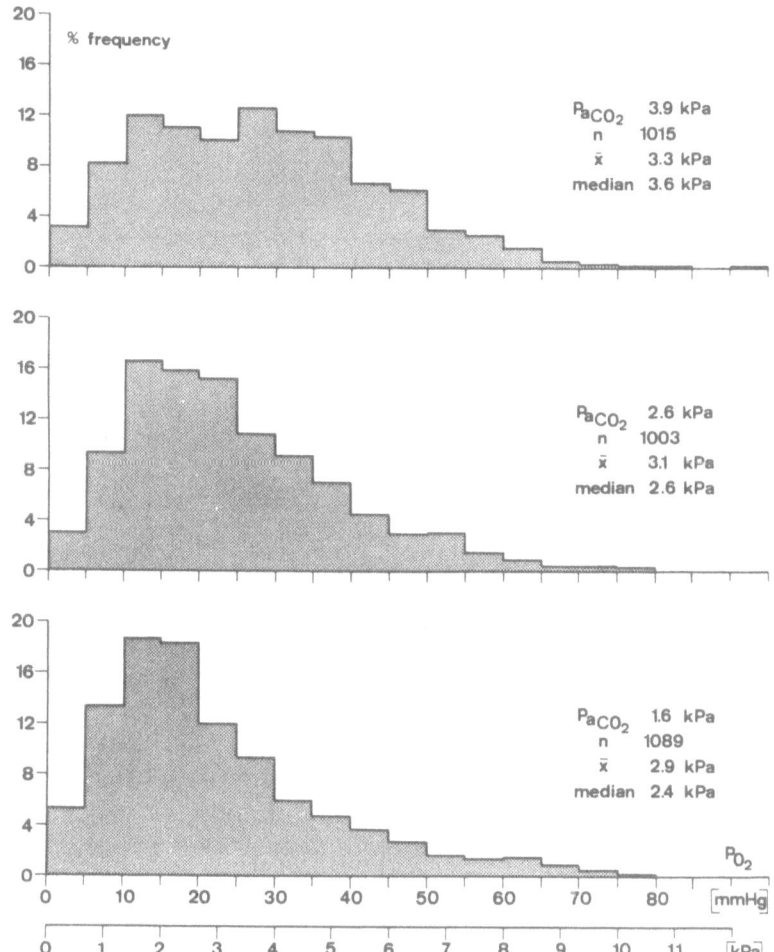

Fig. 2. PO_2 histograms of the brain cortex of cats determined during arterial normocapnia and during arterial hypocapnia ($PaCO_2$ = 19 mmHg and 12 mmHg respectively).

the PO_2 histograms to lower values. Critical oxygen supply conditions for the brain cortex were reached after lowering the arterial CO_2 tension below 15 mmHg (2.0 kPa). As can be seen in Figure 2 the decrease of arterial CO_2 tension to 12 mmHg (1.6 kPa) induced a significant increase in the number of tissue PO_2 values between 0 and 2.5 mmHg (0 - 0.3 kPa) demonstrating the presence of pronounced tissue hypoxia.

At the same time the tissue concentrations of lactate, and pyruvate ratios were found to be significantly above the normal level, which reflects a stimulation of glycolysis (see Table 2). Since in

addition, the phosphocreatine concentration was significantly decreased, insufficient brain cortex oxygen supply must be concluded
from the results of the metabolic assays performed during severe
arterial hypocapnia (Ganholm and Siesjö 1969; Granholm et al., 1969;
Granholm and Siesjö 1971; Grote et al., 1981).

In summary, the above results of tissue PO_2 measurements and
tissue metabolite assays performed in lightly anaesthetized cats
during arterial hypoxia or arterial hypocapnia, demonstrate the
presence of critical oxygen supply conditions in the brain when
arterial O_2 tension was decreased to values of ca. 50 mmHg (6.7 kPa)
and arterial CO_2 tension to ca. 12 mmHg (1.6 kPa), respectively.
Under both conditions a pronounced shift of the tissue PO_2 histograms
to low values and a significant increase in the number of oxygen
tensions between 0 and 2.5 mmHg (0 - 0.3 kPa) was found. Simultaneously, metabolite concentration changes typical for an insufficient tissue O_2 supply were observed. Since during both experimental series brain perfusion pressure reminded normal, elevated
thresholds for critical cerebral O_2 supply during arterial hypoxia
and arterial hypocapnia have to be expected under conditions of
impaired autoregulation of cortical blood flow or pronounced hypotension with mean blood pressure values below ca. 60 mmHg (8.0 kPa).

REFERENCES

Betz, E., 1972, Cerebral blood flow: its measurement and regulation,
    Physiol.Rev., 52:595-630.
Chance, B., Schoener, B., and Schindler, F., 1964, The intracellular
    oxidation-reduction state, in: "Oxygen in the Animal
    Organism," F. Dickens and E. Neil, Pergamon Press, Oxford,
    pp.367-372.
Duffy, T. E., Nelson, S. R., and Lowry, O. H., 1972, Cerebral carbo-
    hydrate metabolism during acute hypoxia and recovery,
    J.Neurochem., 19:959-977.
Granholm, L., and Siesjö, B. K., 1969, The effects of hypercapnia and
    hypocapnia upon cerebrospinal fluid lactate and pyruvate
    concentrations and upon the lactate, pyruvate, ATP, ADP,
    phosphocreatine and creatine concentrations of cat brain
    tissue, Acta Physiol.Scand., 75:257-266.
Granholm, L., Lukjanova, L., and Siesjö, B. K., 1969, The effect of
    marked hyperventilation upon tissue levels of NADH, lactate,
    pyruvate, phosphocreatine and adenosine phosphates of the rat
    brain, Acta Physiol.Scand., 77:179-190.
Granholm, L., and Siesjö, B. K., 1971, The effect of combined respir-
    atory and nonrespiratory alkalosis on energy metabolites and
    acid-base parameters in the rat brain, Acta Physiol.Scand.,
    81:307-314.
Grote, J., 1967, Die Sauerstoffspannung im Gehirngewebe, in: "Hydro-
    dynamik, Elektrolyt- und Säure-Basen-Haushalt im Liquor und
    Nervensystem," G. Kienle, ed., Thieme, Stuttgart, pp.41-50.

Grote, J., 1978, Cerebral blood flow regulation under the conditions
    of arterial hypoxia, in: "The Arterial System," R. D. Bauer
    and R. Busse, eds., Springer, Berlin - Heidelberg - New York,
    pp.209-215.
Grote, J., Zimmer, K., and Schubert, R., 1981, Effects of severe
    arterial hypocapnia on regional blood flow regulation, tissue
    PO$_2$ and metabolism in the brain cortex of cats,
    Pflügers Arch., 391:195-199.
Grote, J., and Schubert, R., 1982, Regulation of cerebral perfusion
    and PO$_2$ in normal and edematous brain tissue, in: "Oxygen
    Transport to Human Tissues," J. A. Loeppky and M. L. Riedesel,
    eds., Elsevier/North-Holland, New York - Amsterdam - Oxford,
    pp.169-178.
Hutten, H., and Brock, M., 1969, The two-minutes-flow-index (TMFI),
    in: "Cerebral Blood Flow, Clinical and Experimental Results,"
    M. Brock, C. Fieschi, D. H. Ingvar, N. A. Lassen, and K.
    Schürmann, eds., Springer, Berlin - Heidelberg - New York,
    pp.19-23.
Kessler, M., and Grunewald, W., 1969, Possibilities of measuring
    oxygen pressure fields in tissue by multiwire platinum elec-
    trodes, Progr.Resp.Res., 3:147-152.
Kuschinsky, W., and Wahl, M., 1978, Local chemical and neurogenic
    regulation of cerebral vascular resistance, Physiol.Rev.,
    58:656-689.
Leniger-Follert, E., Lübbers, D. W., and Wrabetz, W., 1975, Regul-
    ation of local tissue PO$_2$ of brain cortex at different
    arterial O$_2$ pressures, Pflügers Arch., 359:81-95.
Lübbers, D. W., 1973, Local tissue PO$_2$; its measurement and meaning,
    in: "Urban und Schwarzenberg," M. Kessler, D. F. Bruley, L. C.
    Clark, D. W. Lübbers, I. A. Silver, and J. Strauss, eds.,
    München, pp.151-155.
Lübbers, D. W., Baumgärtl, H., Fabel, H., Huch, A., Kessler, M.,
    Kunze, K., Riemann, H., Sieler, D., and Schuchardt, S., 1969,
    Principle and construction of various platinum electrodes,
    Progr.Resp.Res., 3:136-146.
Norberg, K., and Siesjö, B. K., 1975, Cerebral metabolism in hypoxic
    hypoxia. I. Pattern of activation of glycolysis: a reevalu-
    ation, Brain Res., 86:31-44.
Norberg, K., Quistorff, B., and Siesjö, B. K., 1975, Effects of
    hypoxia of 10-45 seconds duration on energy metabolism in the
    cerebral cortex of unanesthetized and anesthetized rats,
    Acta Physiol. Scand., 95:301-310.
Opitz, E., und Schneider, M., 1950, Über die Sauerstoffversorgung des
    Gehirns und den Mechanismus von Mangelwirkungen, Erg.Physiol.,
    46:126-260.
Schmahl, F. W., Betz, E., Dettinger, E., and Hohorst, H. J., 1966,
    Energiestoffwechsel der Großhirnrinde und Elektroencephal-
    ogramm bei Sauerstoffmangel, Pflügers Arch., 292:46-59.
Zierler, K. L., 1965, Equations for measuring blood flow by external
    monitoring of radioisotopes, Circ.Res., 16:309-321.

V

CLINICAL ASPECTS OF CONTROLLED HYPOTENSION

VARIATIONS OF INSTANTANEOUS HEART RATE DURING
NEUROLEPTANESTHESIA WITH CONCOMITANT CONTINUOUS
INFUSIONS OF ALTHESIN AND SODIUM NITROPRUSSIDE

K. Huse and M. Krämer

Department of Anesthesia and
Department of Neurosurgery
University of Düsseldorf, FRG

INTRODUCTION

Althesin is a steroid anesthetic agent for intravenous use. In
this study, Althesin was used in combination for induction and maintenance of anesthesia for neurosurgical procedures. In addition the
patient received sodium nitroprusside for a limited period of controlled hypotension. The particular advantage of Althesin for use
with neurosurgical patients is its moderate hypotensive effect together with a major decrease of intracranial pressure. The study of
Takashi et al. (1973) on all normal persons demonstrated a decrease
of the cerebrospinal fluid pressure by 45% after administration of
Althesin. The decrease of intracranial pressure may be due to the
decrease of intracerebral blood volume. Pickerodt et al. (1972)
observed a 21% carotid blood flow reduction in monkeys after induction of anesthesia with 50 μl/kg Althesin; the CMR_{O_2} of the gray
brain matter decreased by 40%. The value of Nitroprusside for a safe
reduction in blood pressure is well documented in the literature
(Huse 1977, Adams 1973, Page 1955). The special aim of the present
study was to document the response of heart rate in neuroleptanesthesia with concomitant continous medication of Althesin and controlled hypotension with sodium nitroprusside. Instantaneous heart
rate was determined because it is well suited to demonstrate the
pharmacological effects of different drugs on the heart rate.

METHODS

Patients and Clinical Procedure

12 neurosurgical patients were examined. The mean age was 44±6
(range 25-55), the average height was 172±10, weight 77±16 kg. The

patients were premedicated with 0.5 mg Scopolamine, 2.5-5 mg
Droperidol and 25-50 mg Pentobarbital. After arrival in the operating room, anesthesia was induced with Althesin (50 µl/kg) and
maintained with N_2/O_2 and Fentanyl (average total dose 1.74 ±
0.745 mg). In addition the patients received Althesin (average dose:
59.7 ± 43 ml) via continuous infusion of 10-30 ml/h. Controlled
hypotension for a limited time was induced with sodium nitroprusside.

EXPERIMENTAL PROCEDURE

The RR intervals were measured, stored and retrieved by a small,
modular PDP 11 computer system. The configuration is demonstrated in
Figure 1. It consists of a Plessey Peripherals Micro One which is a
DEC LSI 11/02 processor equipped with 64 kbytes of memory,

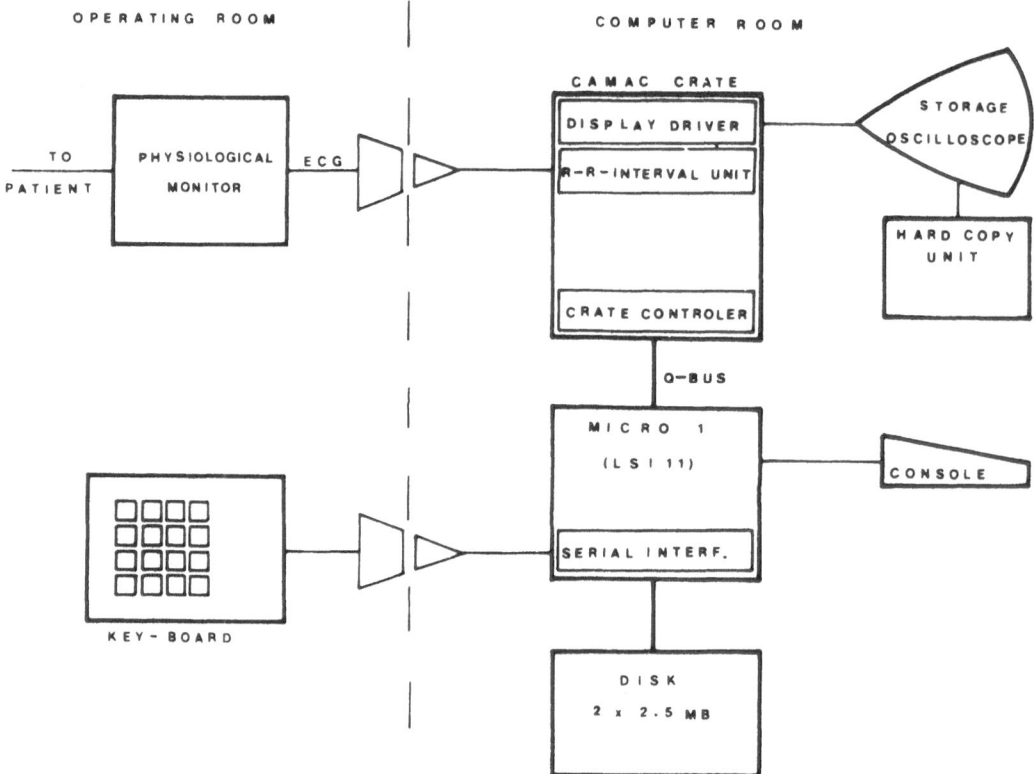

Fig. 1.   System configuration. Right side: computer room with DEC
          LSI 11 Computer, Camac process interface and graphical
          display unit. Left side: operating room, physiological
          monitor for ECG monitoring, function key board for event
          marking. Analog data transmission via isolation amplifier.

and RK 05 compatible disc of two times 2.5 Mbyte capacity. A tele-
type corporation KSR 43 terminal is used for print out and system
control. Event marking is done with a 16 key board in the operating
room via a serial transmission line coupled by an isolation amplifier
and a DL 11 serial interface to the computer. A Camac Crate is used
as compact process interface. It is coupled to the computer with a
Q-Bus cable and a Schlumberger JLSI 10 Single Crate Controler. The
advantage of this modular system is the ease of mixing commercially
available interface units with experimental ones wired and soldered
on prototyping boards. We use a Schlumberger JDD 10 for driving a
Tektronix 411 Storage Oscilloscope and 4601 Hardcopy unit to give
graphical output and documentation.

The RR Intervals are measured with an ECG processing module
which was especially developed and built on a prototyping board.
The ECG of the patient conventionally monitored in the operating
room by a Tektronix Physiological Monitor is transmitted to the
computer room by an analog line and isolation amplifier. After
being fed to the processing unit, the ECG is filtered, amplified,
automatically gain controlled, differentiated and triggered by a
circuit which was developed based on a QRS detector by Winter and
Trendholm (1969). Time between QRS triggers is measured digitally
with a resolution of one millisecond. An interruption causes the
computer to read the interval information, and buffer it in the
memory while storing blocks of 256 intervals in individual patient
records in a large disc file. The word length of the PDP 11 computer
series is 16 bit. A single word can range from $-32,768$ to $+32,767$,
or from zero to 32,767 seconds – implying a resolution of 1 millisecond. Negative values for RR intervals are not possible, with the
exception that we use negative values to mark a missing QRS trigger.
The hardware send an interrupt at least every 8.192 seconds which
avoids an overflow condition and lost time synchronization in the
case of very large intervals due to physiologic reasons or artifacts.
The disc file consists of 4500 random access data blocks. The first
block contains the file directory. The records of this organization
block are described by record numbers and pointers to the beginning
and end of each record. At the beginning of each record one block
contains additional information such as actual date and time of the
observation period, patient name, and a data field with type, time
and position (block number and number of intervals in the block) of
event marks. The event marks are generated by pressing a button on
the keyboard in the operating room. The data is stored on-line and
retrieved off-line by a set of specially developed programs.

RESULTS

The results of this study are summarized in Table 1 and
Figures 2-5.

DISCUSSION

The chronotropic effect of different agents can be of different origin. First we have to consider the direct action on the myocardium, then the effect on the autonomic regulation. The autonomic equilibrium can be disturbed by different mechanisms.

1. Reflex mechanisms
2. Central nervous mechanisms
3. Peripheral mechanisms
4. Ganglionic action, adrenergic receptors, cholinergic receptors

Althesin and Fentanyl have the following effects:

Sympathetic activity	Vagal activity
Fentanyl ↑	(Central vagal activation) ↑
Althesin ↓	(Central vagal inhibition) ↓

The bradycardia after application of Fentanyl is due to central vagal activation. According to the study of Arndt et al. (1980), sympathetic activity remains unchanged after fentanyl medication. The maximal activity is reached when all the opiate receptors are saturated. Parallel to the effect of Fentanyl on the cardioinhibitory vagal centers, a negative chromotropic effect on the heart rate can be demonstrated. The receptors are saturated when an additional dose will not augment the negative chronotropic effect, and thus a plateau of persistent bradycardia can be demonstrated (Figures 2, 3, 4, 5).

Table 1. Mean Heart Rate (f) and Mean RR Intervals (MS) of 12 Patients.

	Heart rate (beat/min)	RR interval (MS)
Preoperative control	68 ± 12	994 ± 165
Induction of anesthesia	81 ± 13	830 ± 130
Neuroleptanesthesia	55 ± 8	1115 ± 139
Continuous infusion of Althesin	73 ± 9	837 ± 105
Controlled hypotension with Sodium nitroprusside	85 ± 20	752 ± 168

Significance

1 vs. 2	$p < 0.02$ significant	3 vs. 1	$p < 0.01$ significant
1 vs. 3	$p < 0.01$ significant	3 vs. 2	$p < 0.001$ significant
1 vs. 4	$p > 0.05$ nonsignificant	3 vs. 4	$p < 0.001$ significant
1 vs. 5	$p < 0.02$ significant	3 vs. 5	$p < 0.001$ significant

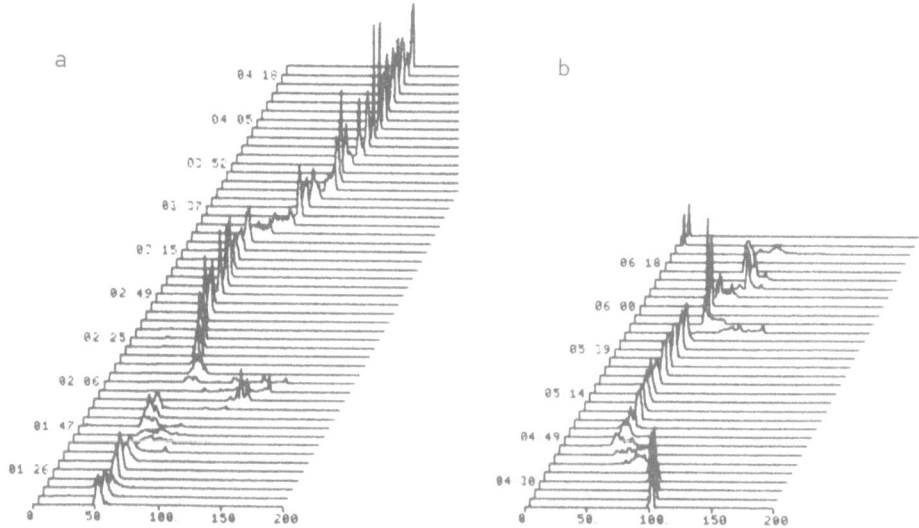

Fig. 2.   Frequency distribution curve of heart rate. Horizontal
         axis: heart rate (beats/min), vertical axis: time axis
         (min). Preoperative phase (01.26) (numbers represent hours
         and minutes respectively). Induction of anesthesia with
         Althesin (02.06). Neuroleptanesthesia and continuous
         infusion of Althesin (03.37). Controlled hypotension with
         Sodium nitroprusside (04.30). Extubation (06.18).

     Different authors described an increase in heart rate of 14-20%
after application of Althesin (Cohen et al., 1973; Sonntag el at.,
1973; Tammisto et al., 1973; Savege 1973). The positive chronotropic
effect of Althesin is due to vagal inhibition. This effect is partially antagonized by central activation of Fentanyl, and thus
Althesin application during neuroleptanesthesia produces only a
moderate increase in heart rate.

     During neuroleptanesthesia and continuous infusion of Althesin,
controlled hypotension with sodium nitroprusside initiated further
cardioacceleration. The studies of Page et al. (1955) dismissed any
central effect of sodium nitroprusside. This additional chronotropic
effect can only be explained as a peripheral reflex mechanism, since
neuroleptanesthesia does not inhibit the baroreceptor reflex (Arndt
et al., 1980; Inoue et al., 1980). Besides the effect on heart rate,
Althesin has a moderate hypotensive effect that reduces the total
dose of sodium nitroprussde and assures smooth controlled hypotension
and prevents posthypotensive reactive hypertension.

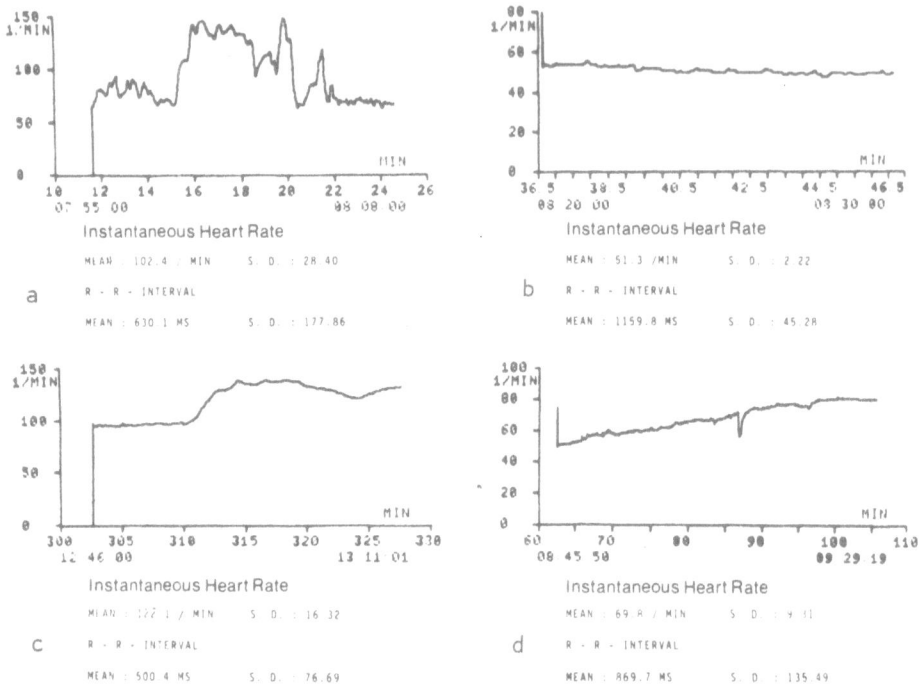

Fig. 3.   x-axis: time (min); y-axis: instantaneous heart rate (f).
a) Induction of anesthesia with Althesin. The average preoperative instantaneous heart rate was 76 ± 7. After injection of Althesin, sudden increase of the instantaneous
heart rate and return to the original level after 5 min.
b) Plateau formation of the instantaneous heart rate with
minimal variations of the instantaneous heart rate in neuroleptanesthesia and controlled respiration. c) Increase of
the heart rate from 51 ± 2 to 122 ± 16 after induction of
controlled hypotension with sodium nitroprusside to 122 ±·
16. d) Moderate slow increase of the instantaneous heart
rate after continuous infusion of Althesin.

SUMMARY

     In 12 neurosurgical patients with cerebral aneurysm, ECG was
monitored in the operating room. The ECG was transmitted to the
computer room and RR intervals were measured on-line and stored by a
hardware QRS detector connected to a PDP 11 computer system. Soft-
ware was available to analyze the data. The following methods were
used: trend plotting, frequency distribution, scatter diagrams and
standard statistical analysis.

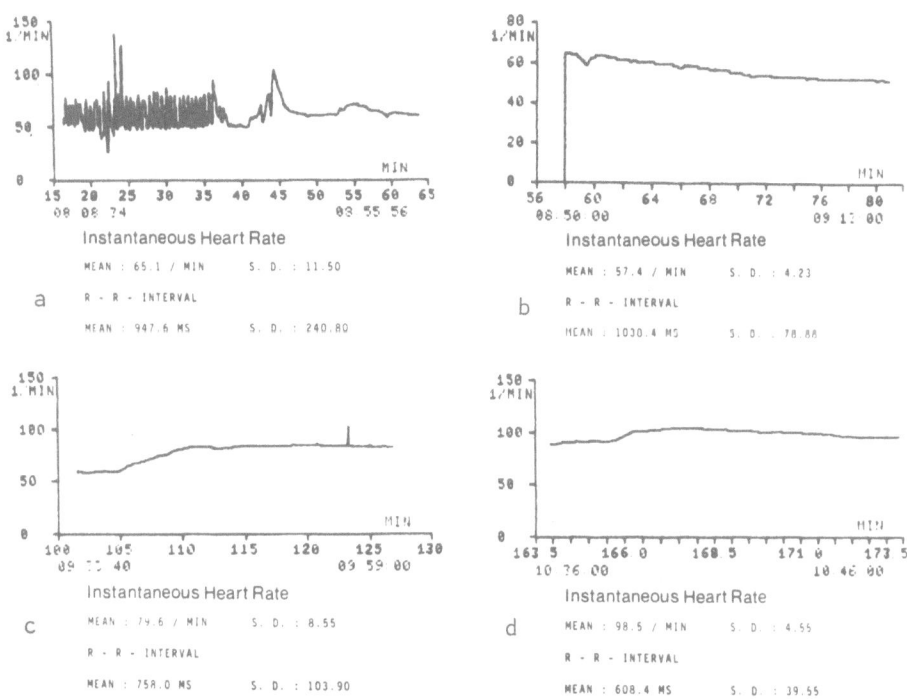

Fig. 4. x-axis: time (min); y-axis: heart rate (f). a) Instantaneous heart rate of a patient with spontaneous respiration
and a distinct respiratory synchronous dysrhythmia of the
instantaneous heart rate. After induction of anesthesia
(08:38:00) (numbers represent hours, minutes, and seconds
respectively) and controlled respiration, the instantaneous
heart rate shows minimal variations. b) Bradycardia in
neuroleptanesthesia due to the central vagal activation
by fentanyl. c) Due to the central vagolytic action of
Althesin, an increase in instantaneous heart rate from
57 ± 4 to 80 ±·8 after continuous infusion of Althesin.
After a time interval during constant dose of Althesin,
a plateau form of the instantaneous heart rate can be observed. d) Moderate increase of the instantaneous heart
rate from a mean value of 80 ± 3 to 99 ± 4 during sodium
nitroprusside infusion.

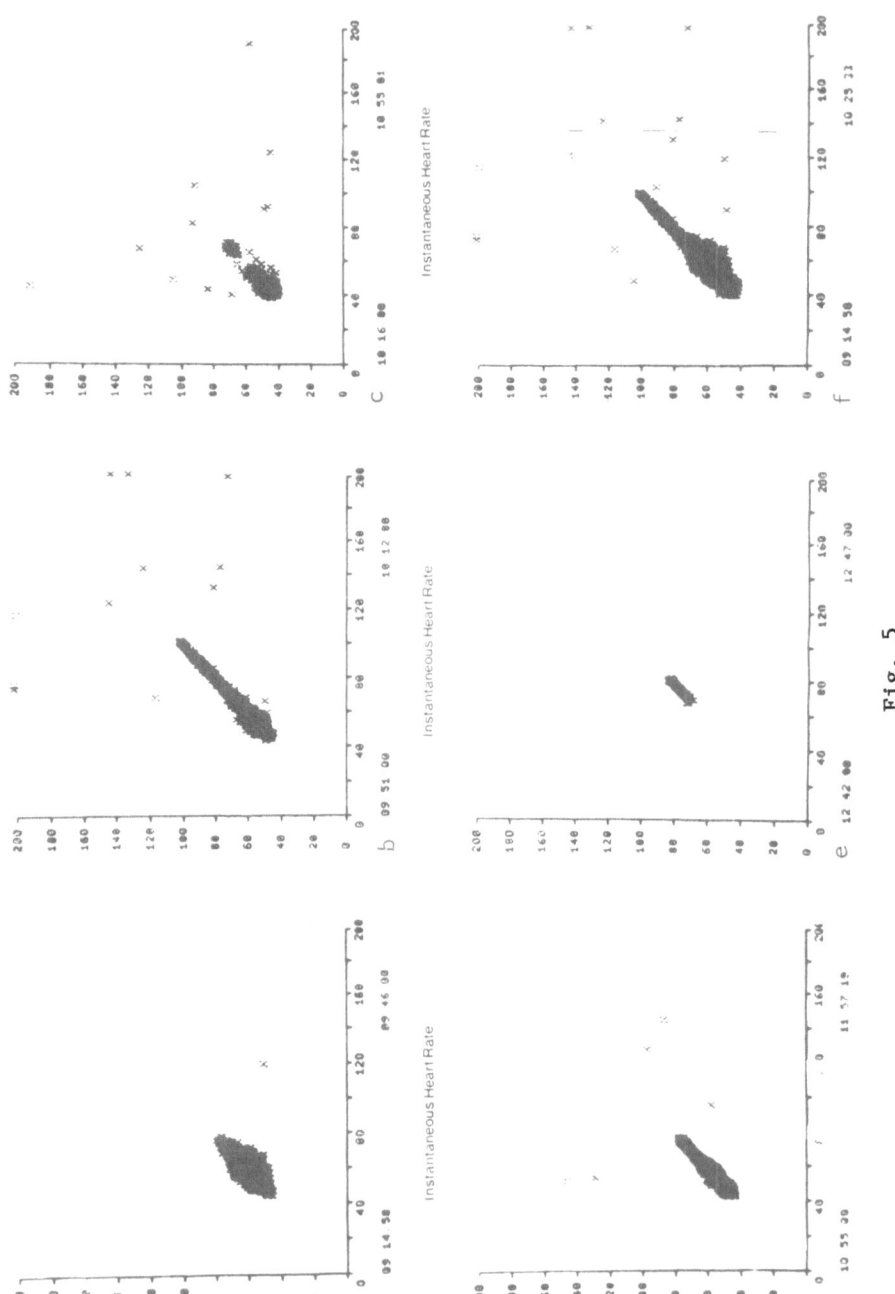

Fig. 5

Fig. 5. x-axis: time (min); y-axis: RR interval. a) Distribution of
the preoperative scattergram. b) Scattergram of the induction period of anesthesia after application of Althesin.
The shape of the scattergram shows the temporary tachycardia
after injection of Althesin. c) Scattergram of the instantaneous heart rate during neuroleptanesthesia and continuous
infusion of Althesin. d) Scattergram during neuroleptanesthesia and continuous infusion of Althesin. e) Scattergram
during neuroleptanesthesia and controlled hypotension with
sodium nitroprusside. f) Scattergram of the instantaneous
heart rate during and after controlled hypotension with
sodium nitroprusside.

REFERENCES

Arndt, J. O., and Mameghami, F., 1980, Die Funktion homöostatischer
    Kreislaufreflexe unter Etomidate, Fentanyl und Dehydrobenz-
    peridol, Anaesthesist, 29:200.
Cohen, R. S., Creighton, R. E., Nisbet, H. J. A., McDonald, P., and
    Steward, D. J., 1973, The effects of Althesin on cerebral
    blood flow and intracranial pressure, Canad.Anaesth.Soc.J.,
    754.
Cohen, R. S., Nisbet, H. J. A., Creighton, R. E., Steward, D. J., and
    McDonald, P., 1973, The effect of hypoxaemia on cerebral blood
    flow and cerebrospinal fluid pressure in dogs anaesthetized
    with Althesin, Pentobarbitone and Methoxyflurane, Canad.
    Anaesth.Soc.J., 20:757.
Du Cailar, J., 1972, The effects in man of infusions of Althesin
    with particular regard to the cardiovascular system,
    Postgraduate Med.J. (June Suppl.).
Coleman, A. J., Downing, J. W., Leary, W. P., Moyes, D. G., and
    Styles, M., 1972, The immediate cardiovascular effects of
    Althesin (Glaxo CT 1341), a steroid induction agent, and
    thiopental in man, Anethesia, 27:373 (1972).
Campbell, D., Forreser, A. C., Miller, D. C., Hutton, J. A., Kennedy,
    J. A., Lawrie, T. D. V., Lorimer, A. R., and McCall, D., 1971,
    A preliminary clinical study of CT 1341 - a steroid anaes-
    thetic agent, Brit.J.Anaesth., 43:14.
Harrison, S. G. C., and Sellick, B. A., 1972, Cardiovascular effects
    of Althesin in patients with cardiac pathology. Preliminary
    communication, Brit.J.Anaesth., 44:1205.
Huse, K., 1977, Kie kontrollierte hypotension mit nitroprussidnatrium
    in der neuroanaesthesie, in: "Anaesthesiologie und Wiederbele-
    bung," B. 107, R. Frey, F. Kern, and O. Mayrhofer, Hrsg.,
    Springer Verlag, Berlin - Heidelberg - New York.
Inoue, K., Samodele, L. F., and Arndt, J. O., 1980, Fentanyl
    activates a particular population of vagal efferents which are
    cardioinhibitory, Naunyn-Schmiedeberg's Arch.Pharmacol.,
    312:57.

Miller, D. C., Bradford, E. M. W., and Campbell, D., 1972, Haemo-
    dynamic effects of Althesin in poor-risk patients,
    Postgraduate Med.J. (June Suppl.).
Page, J. H., Corcoran, A. C., Dustan, H. P., and Koppany, T., 1955,
    Cardiovascular actions of sodium nitroprusside in animals and
    hypotensive patients, Circulation, 11:188.
Pickerodt, V. W. A., McDowall, D. G., Coroneos, N. J., and Keaney,
    N. P., 1972, Effect of Althesin on cerebral perfusion, cere-
    bral metabolism and intracranial pressure in the anaesthes-
    tized baboon, Brit.J.Anaesth., 44:751.
Patschke, D., Brückner, J. B., Reinecke, A., Schmicke, P., Tarnow,
    J., and Eberlein, H., 1972, Experimental investigations on the
    circulatory effects of CT 1341, a new steroid anaesthetic,
    Der Anaesthesist, 21:338.
Sonntag, H., Schenk, H. D., Regensburger, D., Kettler, D., Hellberg,
    K., Knoll, D., Donath, U., and Becker, H., 1973, Effects of
    Althesin (Glaxo CT 1341) on coronary blood flow and myocardial
    metabolism in man, Acta Anaesthesiol.Scand., 17:(4) 218.
Tammisto, T., Takki, S., Tigerstedt, J., and Kanste, A., 1973, A
    comparison of Althesin and thiopental in induction of anaes-
    thesia, Brit.J.Anaesth., 45:100.
Takahashi, T., Takasaki, M., Namik, A., and Dolvi, S., 1973, Effects
    of Althesin on cerebrospinal fluid pressure, Brit.J.Anaesth.,
    45:179.
Turner, J. M., Coroneos, N. J., Gibson, R. M., Powell, D., Ness,
    M. A., and McDowall, D. G., 1973, The effect of Althesin on
    intracranial pressure in man, Brit.J.Anaesth., 45:168.
Savege, T. M., Blogg, C. E., Foley, E. J., Ross, L., Lang, M., and
    Simpson, B. R., 1973, The cardiorespiratory effects of
    Althesin and Ketamine. A comparison, Anaesthesia, 28:391.
Savege, T. M., Foley, E. I., Coultas, R. J., Walton, B., Strumin, C.,
    and Simpson, B. R., 1973, The cardiorespiratory effects of
    Althesin and Ketamine. A comparison, Anaesthesia, 28:391.
Savege, T. M., Foley, E. I., Coultas, R. J., Walton, B., Strumin, C.,
    Simpson, B. R., and Scott, D. F., 1971, CT 1341 Some effects
    in men. Cardiorespiratory electroencephalography and bio-
    chemical measurements, Brit.J.Anaesth., 26:402.

LIMITATIONS OF INDUCED HYPOTENSION

U. Braun, J. Jansen, G. Rahlf and E. Turner

Department of Anesthesiology, Department of Pathology
and Department of Neurosurgery
University of Göttingen, FRG

Induced hypotension today is a well established technique. It
is clear though, that manipulating blood pressure is a delicate
issue. Every anaesthetist who deals with it should know the limitations and complications of the methods. In this paper we would
like to deal with some fundamentals of blood pressure, organ perfusion and tissue oxygenation followed by a case report. We shall
end with some considerations for the clinical management of induced
hypotension.

SOME FUNDAMENTALS OF BLOOD PRESSURE, ORGAN PERFUSION AND TISSUE OXYGENATION

By analogy with Ohm's law the pressure drop is related to blood
flow and resistance ($\Delta P = F \cdot R$). Resistance depends upon the nature
of the fluid and the geometric dimensions of the vessels. Induction
of hypotension can only leave flow constant, if resistance is reduced. In case of unchanged resistance flow decreases. This is not
only true for the whole organism, but also for any perfused organ.
The measurement of blood pressure per se offers no information concerning blood flow, flow distribution or oxygen supply of the tissues. Inducing hypotension for bloodless operating field and reduction of blood loss is a practical approach with no strict rationale.
The margin of safety for the patient is reduced and the efforts of
the anaesthetist must be greatly enlarged.

Complications cannot be avoided with certainty by the closest
monitoring of intravascular pressure, if that pressure happens to be
inadequate for a particular patient (Lindop 1975; Prys-Roberts et
al., 1974).

Another fundamental relation is the Fick principle. (Flow equals the ratio of O_2-uptake and a-v oxygen content difference). If flow is decreased by deliberate hypotension and oxygen consumption remains constant, central venous oxygen saturation is diminished. This may be harmful for tissue oxygenation. If O_2-uptake is reduced, this may reflect a perfusion deficit. It is useful to remember, that sufficient arterial oxygenation alone cannot guarantee safe tissue oxygen supply. Measurements of O_2-uptake ($\dot{V}O_2$) indicate that there is decrease of $\dot{V}O_2$ during hypotension (Kalff and Schäfer 1970). This can be confirmed by our own observations. For the clinical situation this seems to be tolerable although further investigation is needed because both drug application (for example barbiturates) and hyperventilation are not without influence upon $\dot{V}O_2$.

Hyperventilation is often used together with deliberate hypotension. Our own findings suggest that hyperventilation has a metabolic effect (increase in $\dot{V}O_2$) in neurosurgical patients, which is met by an increased arterio-venous oxygen content difference (Figure 1, 2). This observation, which suggests detrimental effects in cardiovascular patients, leads us to conclude that some of the aspects of controlled hypotension that are valuable practically, have not been fully investigated.

Autoregulation of vital organs offers some independence from the systemic circulation. The metabolic demands of the brain are rather constant under conditions of health. Cerebral perfusion is influenced by arterial pCO_2, pO_2, anaesthetics, hypotensive drugs and temperature. Autoregulation is lost during severe hypotension, hypoxemia, acidosis, increased intracranial pressure and occlusive cerebro-vascular disease.

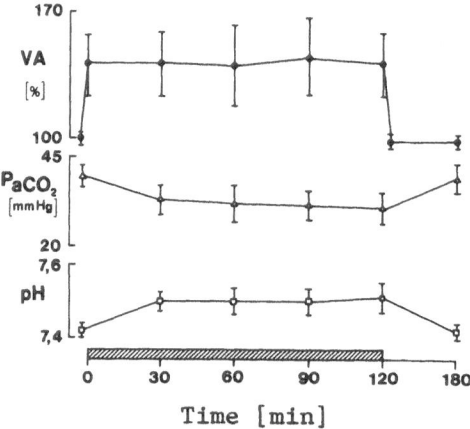

Fig. 1. Hyperventilation in 10 neurosurgical patients. The respiratory rate was increased from 10 to 14/min for 2 hours. Alveolar ventilation ($\dot{V}A$) was increased by 40%.

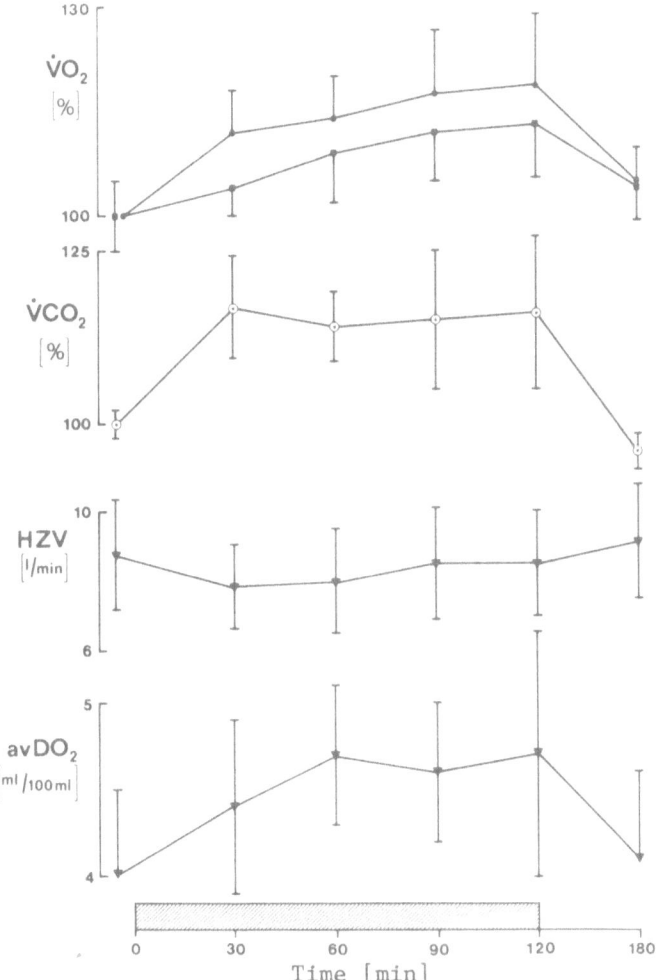

Fig. 2.   The effect of hyperventilation on $\dot{V}O_2$, $\dot{V}CO_2$, cardiac output
          (HZV) and arterio-venous oxygen content difference. VO_2 was
          measured with two different methods (cardiac output plus
          oxygen analysis in arterial and venous blood and a non-
          invasive technique (Braun et al., 1980; Braun et al., 1982),
          which yielded higher results).

     For the management of deliberate hypotension it is important to
know that there may be some cerebral regions with intact and others
with lost autoregulation and that therapeutic steps are taken to
secure tissue oxygenation in those regions with lost autoregulation.
It cannot be denied though that our assumptions are hypothetical and
that no means of controlling regional cerebral well-being are at
hand. Perfusion of the heart, which also shows some autoregulative

capability, is subject to the metabolic demands of the organ. These
are closely related to the mechanical action of the organ. For example wall tension, contractility and heart rate have large oxygen
cost and therefore strong influence upon coronary blood flow. Basal
metabolism and activation energy have little influence. During sys-
tole there is no coronary blood flow. Variations of cardiac O_2-
demands must be met by the coronary circulation, for which the mean
diastolic value is the driving pressure. As for coronary heart
disease, decreased perfusion pressure in deliberate hypotension combined with increased heart rate may be responsible for an imbalance
of O_2-supply and -demand. In patients with congestive heart disease
and hypertension, reduced coronary perfusion may also be deleterious.
Arterial pCO_2, choice of anaesthetic and the surgical conditions are
also not without influence upon the coronary circulation. Autoregulation of the kidney is not maintained during anaesthesia. Reduction
of RBF and GFR can be attributed to anaesthesia and of course deliberate hypotension, but no serious complications may result for the
kidney. The same is true for the liver, which is subject to all
changing systemic circulatory conditions. An important funtional
change of the lung is the increase in physiologic deadspace by reduction of perfusion.

CASE REPORT

     In 1978 a 49-year-old male patient was scheduled for clipping of
a cerebral aneurysm in our clinic in Göttingen. He had no history of
cardiac disease and his clinical examination revealed no gross abnormalities (Figure 3, 4). Hypotension was induced with halothane. The
mean arterial pressure was slowly reduced to 80 mmHg (invasive measurement). Suddenly, before the clipping could be started, there was
a pressure drop to a mean value of 50 mmHg followed by a sudden
cardiac arrest. All attempts at resuscitation were without success.
Pathology revealed coronary artery disease (CAD): arteriosclerotic
disease of all branches of the coronary system, almost complete
stenosis of the Ramus interventricularis (Figure 5) and 80% stenosis
of the Ramus circumflexus of the left artery.

     It is remarkable to hear that the patient had no history of CAD,
but this feature is not unusual. According to an American review
(Lown 1979) there is a large incidence of sudden cardiac death (SCD)
among all fatalities of ischemic heart disease. Nearly 25% of persons dying suddenly have had no prior recognized symptoms of heart
disease. This adds up to a number of approximately 100,000 fatalities of SCD in the U.S.A. per year (Germany about 15,000) without a
known history of CAD. There is no doubt that controlled hypotension
is a threat to life in a patient with CAD. Even with very careful
history taking and thorough preoperative evaluation there remains
lack of confidence that it is possible to exclude all CAD patients
from hypotension.

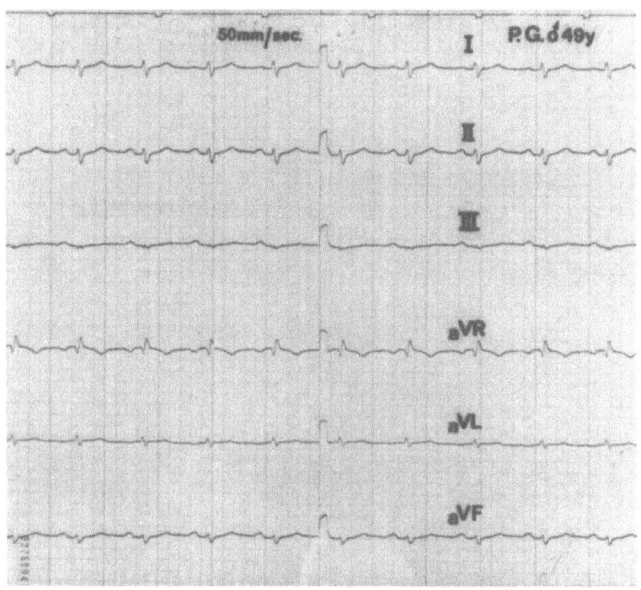

Fig. 3.   Preoperative electrocardiogram: I, II, III, aVR, aVL, aVF.

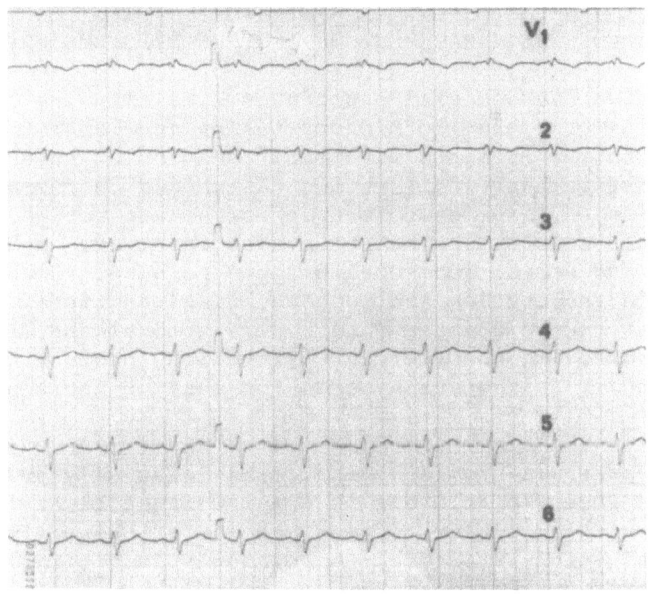

Fig. 4.   Preoperative electrocardiogram: V_1-V_6.

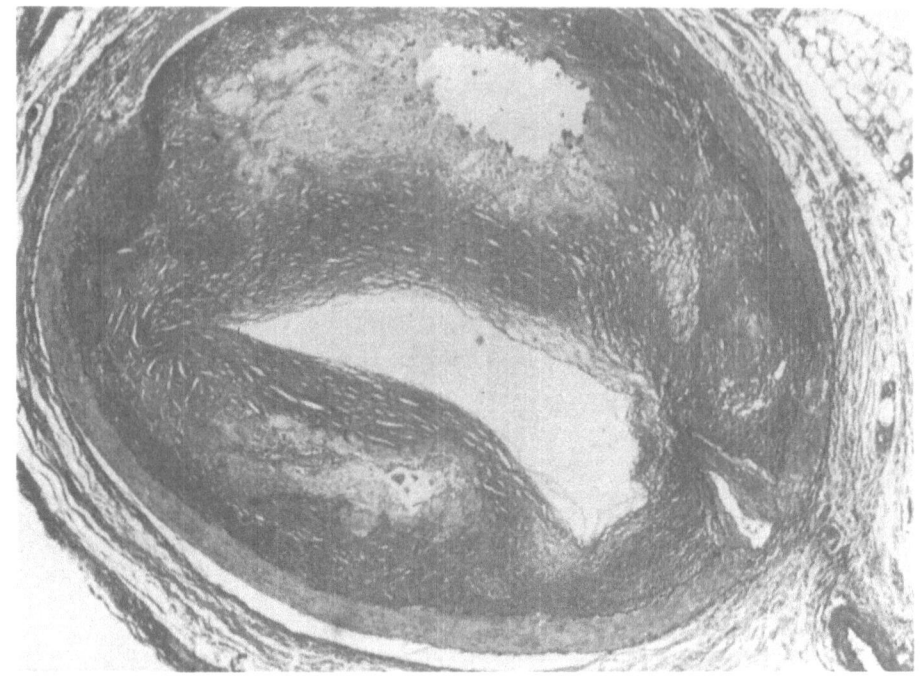

Fig. 5.   Ramus interventricularis of the left coronary artery, almost
           complete stenosis.

CONSIDERATIONS FOR THE MANAGEMENT OF INDUCED HYPOTENSION.

        For elective neurosurgial procedures like clipping of an aneur-
ysm very careful preoperative history taking and laboratory evaluation is mandatory. Patients with manifestation of cerebro-vascular
disease, congestive heart failure and CAD should be discarded from
induced hypotension. The same is true for severe peripheral vascular
disease, because usually the heart is also involved. β-Blockade 3
days prior to and during anaesthesia seems to be of value to cope
with adverse intraoperative and postoperative reactions. The hypertensive patient can be treated with a very gradual and mild reduction
of blood pressure. In the emergency situation (profuse bleeding)
the indication for deliberate hypotension must be treated more
generously.

        Arterial pressure should be monitored invasively or with in-
direct methods that are reliable in the low range also. Invasive
measurement, which we prefer, offers access for the analysis of blood
gases. Central venous pressure, temperature and expired CO_2 should
also be monitored. Precordial ECG leads and cerebral function monitor (CFM) must be advocated for cardial and cerebral organ control,
but both methods have limited value for the early detection of de-

leterious events. In our institute the placement of a Swan-Ganz
catheter is a routine procedure for several clinical situations such
as deliberate hypotension. Apart from the possibility of flow measurement, PAP and central venous O_2-saturation can be measured. With
improved facilities in the future it might be of benefit to have
continuous noninvasive values of $\dot{V}O_2$ and $\dot{V}CO_2$ (Braun et al., 1980;
Braun et al., 1982. 1982).

REFERENCES

Braun, U., Turner, E., and Freiboth, K., 1980, Continuous monitoring
        of oxygen uptake and carbon dioxide elimination in critically
        ill patients. International Congress Series No. 538, p.665,
        "Anesthesiology, Proceedings of the 7th World Congress of
        Anaesthesiologists," Hamburg, Sept.14-21, ISBN Excerpta
        Medica, Amsterdam - Oxford - Princeton.
Braun, U., Turner, E., and Freiboth, K., 1982, Ein Verfahren zur
        Bestimmung von O_2-Aufnahme und CO_2-Abgabe aus den Atemgasen
        beim beatmeten Patienten, Anaesthesist, 31 (in press).
Kalff, G., and Schäfer, E. D., 1970, Influence of controlled hypo-
        tension on body-oxygen consumption, Acta anaesth.Scand.,
        Suppl.XXXVII, 152.
Lindop, M. J., 1975, Complications and morbidity of controlled hypo-
        tension, Brit.J.Anaesth., 47:799.
Lown, B., 1979, Sudden cardiac death: the major challenge confronting
        contemporary cardiology, Amer.J.Card., 43:313.
Prys-Roberts, C., Lloyd, J. W., Fisher, A., Kerr, J. H., and
        Patterson, T. J. H., 1974, Deliberate profound hypotension
        induced with halothane, Brit.J.Anaesth., 46:105.

PRO AND CONTRA HYPOTENSION IN NEUROSURGERY

E. Gordon

Department of Anesthesia
Karolinska Hospital
104 01 Stockholm, Sweden

INTRODUCTION

From the beginning of the practice of modern anaesthesia, established procedure demanded the maintenance of normal arterial pressure. The early reports at the end of the 40's that hypotension is
not only innocuous but in some instances even beneficial was met with
astonished incredulity and suspicion by many anaesthetists. And even
if a great portion of this incredulity has vanished since then, some
of the prejudice against the technique of controlled hypotension (CH)
still remains.

In clinical practice there is need for constant review of the
balance of benefits associated with various therapeutic interventions, and their disadvantages. These drawbacks must include not
only the actual hazards of treatment but the more subtle consequences
of depriving the patient of the ability to cope with the hazards of
anaesthesia and operation, and to react to these stresses in a normal
physiological way. With these needs in mind it is somewhat disturb-
ing to realize that much of the current use of the technique of
controlled hypotension is based upon empirical observations even if
it is supported by reasonable explanations. It is questionable
whether such gross observations can be correctly interpreted as few
of the many clinically relevant physiological or pathological re-
lationships have been sufficiently defined to allow accurate infer-
ence of cause or effect. A certain mean arterial pressure, for
example, may be necessary to perfuse ischaemic brain tissue, but may
simultaneously increase oedema formation in another region of that
patient's brain. In a third region this perfusion may still be
insufficient to maintain adequate metabolism. The unpredictability
of the consequences of such different effects have to lead either to

the application of more objective monitoring devices or otherwise the
clinician is obliged to perform treatment on extremely unsafe empirical ground, when the clinical outcome will always be uncertain.

It is common knowledge that anaesthetic agents and techniques as
well as even the simplest surgical intervention are a potential risk
for the patient. In performing anaesthesia it is our firm obligation
to remain as close as possible to normal physiology and use drugs and
techniques which cause the least harm to the patient.

There is no disagreement among surgeons and anaesthetists that
CH adds an additional risk to those already inherent in anaesthesia
and operation. These risks are further accentuated in patients where
vital organ systems are already affected preoperatively. It is
therefore of utmost importance that the pros and cons of hypotension
are thoroughly considered in every case before operation, and it
should not be used unless the advantages of the technique exceed its
risks. In the great majority of cases surgeons and anaesthetists
readily agree on the method to be employed in the individual case.
However, in the few cases where such an agreement cannot be reached,
the opinion of the anaesthetist should prevail as he is solely responsible for the selection and use of the different anaesthetic
agents and techniques.

INDICATIONS IN NEUROSURGERY

The indications for CH at the Karolinska Hospital, Stockholm,
have been considerably reduced during the last 10 years, as it is now
used almost exclusively during aneurysm surgery and sometimes during
the removel of arterio-venous malformations. For the removal of
meningiomas or other richly vascularized tumors CH is never used.
The following discussion is therefore based on our experiences during
aneurysm surgery.

The advantage of CH in this field of neurosurgery has been
claimed to be a slackness of the aneurysmal sack making manipulation
during dissection and ligation much easier and diminishing the risk
of rupture. Furthermore, if rupture occurs, bleeding is less tor-
rential and is easier to stem. Studies comparing surgical treatment
of aneurysms with and without CH are rather scarce. One publication
on this subject (Dahlgren et al., 1970) shows that the frequency of
aneurysm rupture is the same whether normotension or hypotension has
been used during surgery. However, agreement among neurosurgeons on
the advantages and the necessity for hypotension during aneurysm
surgery is not universal, nor is there any agreement on the level of
hypotension for the ligation. In many centers surgical treatment of
aneurysms is performed under normotension with practically the same
results as in other clinics where CH is a routine procedure. The
same is valid for the individual cases within the same clinic, and

many patients are operated on successfully under normotension if
circumstances oblige the surgical-anaesthesiogical team to avoid
hypotension for any reason. The reason for these discrepancies are
difficult to analyze. Some of them can be certainly explained by the
varying experience, skillfulness and temperament of the individual
surgeons and perhaps also of the anaesthetists. Others can be rooted
in the traditions of the various institutions and clinics.

CEREBRAL BLOOD FLOW

     In a recent review Lassen (1980) expresses the opinion that in
patients in whom the disease or the surgical intervention has impaired circulation, hypotension is the most effective means of
severely compromising tissue perfusion. This statement is certainly
true in a general sense. On the other hand, it is now fully ap-
preciated that among the vital organs which are most liable to suffer
from the consequences of CH, the brain, and to a lesser degree the
heart, occupy a special place. The great vulnerability of the brain
during hypotension is of vital importance to all clinicians using
this technique. For neurosurgeons and neuroanaesthetists it has
still a more marked relevance, as cerebral circulation and metabolism
are in most cases already in jeopardy before the artificial lowering
of blood pressure.

     When considering the effects of hypotension on the perfusion of
the brain and other vital organs and in trying to define a safe lower
limit of arterial pressure it became evident that no fixed pressure
value can be regarded as optimal for all tissues, as situations are
very different not only in various organs but also in different
regions of the same organ. This applies, of course, even more to the
brain, and especially to the diseased brain, which is most sensitive
to hypoxia and ischaemia.

     Cerebral blood flow (CBF) normally sustains normal neuronal
function if mean cerebral perfusion pressure is maintained over
30 mmHg. However, normal values of total CBF may be misleading and
actually inadequate for several reasons. Firstly, in spite of its
outwardly homogeneous appearance, the normal brain is markedly inhomogeneous both anatomically and physiologically in terms of blood
flow and metablism. Secondly, total CBF may be normal at a time when
regional maldistribution of blood flow, due to hyperperfusion in some
areas and hypoperfusion in others, is occuring. In pathological
states, therefore, it is the regional conditions and not the global
measurements that determine neuronal survival.

REGIONAL BLOOD FLOW

     On the regional level it is possible to define critical thres-
holds of blood flow quite accurately. It was shown both in experi-

mental studies (Branston et al., 1974) and in lightly anaesthetized
humans (Trojaborg and Boysen, 1973; Sundt et al., 1974) that the EEG
and cortical evoked potentials start to decline when CBF drops below
20 ml/100g/min. Below this ischaemic threshold of cortical electric
silence, there is a further ischaemic threshold of metabolic failure
at a flow of about 8-10 ml/100g/min, below which a marked decrease in
tissue ATP occurs, together with a massive release of intracellular
K$^+$ (Astrup et al., 1977). Between these 2 levels there is a
"penumbral" zone somewhere between 15-20 ml/100g/min during prolonged
ischaemia, in which tissue oxygenation is inadequate to sustain
normal function but yet sufficient for the cells to survive (Lassen
and Shapiro, 1981). It is not yet known how often such a "penumbral"
- between life and death - state arises with a reversible ischaemic
paralysis of the neurons. That the state does exist is suggested by
the numerous cases of more or less reversible focal ischaemic lesions
which may last hours, days or perhaps longer, producing varying
extents of neurological deficits in operated patients, and which show
a tendency to a successive clinical improvement.

Hypotension is only one state in which cerebral ischaemia can be
expected. If it is "penumbral" then the level and the duration of
hypotension may determine if symptom remission or cell death will
occur. Other factors that might disrupt the normal balance between
flow and metabolism are loss of autoregulation, vasospasm, and damage
to the blood-brain barrier, cellular oedema, and obstruction of
normal CSF pathways. If we could accurately measure in such clinical
situations the reduced regional flows, or even better, regional
cerebral metabolism, then it would be possible to have much safer
guidelines for the conduct of controlled hypotension. At present
this is impossible, and we do not know in any given patient whether a
given perfusion pressure is adequate to meet the metabolic demands in
all parts of the brain. The positron-emmission CT scanners currently
being developed may make such measurements possible.

EVOKED POTENTIALS

Another possible method of obtaining immediate information concerning the functional state of the brain is the use of electrical
monitoring of cerebral function which has been described in detail
during this symposium (Symon, McDowall, Prior 1981). These reports
suggest a good correlation between the pattern of EEG, evoked response and CFM on the one hand and the degree of neurological dys-
function on the other and may well indicate early changes in cerebral
function in association with decreases in CBF and CPP. However, the
use of these monitoring techniques in the operating theatre is really
in its infancy and it will probably take some time before these techniques are used routinely in every clinic whenever CG is performed.

THE PRESENT CLINICAL SITUATION

Thus, although our knowledge of cerebral circulation and meta-blism during normal and pathological conditions has been greatly improved during recent years, the clinicians who have to decide on the different methods of treatment must still base decisions mainly on empirical grounds. In this respect there are 2 categories of neurosurgeons as far as CH is concerned. One category takes a cautious and restrictive attitude towards CH and is able to perform surgery at normal or moderately lowered levels of blood pressure. The other group of surgeons regard profound hypotension as an absol-ute necessity for performing certain elective surgery and dismiss the risks and dangers of hypotension as belonging exclusively to the theoretical world of laboratories.

The explanation for this descrepancy of views lies not entirely in the differing opinions of clinicians, but also in the extreme difficulty in correlating successive clinical symptoms to the various phases of therapy. Several authors (Brierly and Cooper, 1962; Adams et al., 1966; Fein 1975) have raised, on theoretical grounds, serious objections to induced hypotension. But in the clinical situation, it has been extremely difficult, if not impossible to separate the effects of neurosurgical treatment from the effects of hypotension. Moreover - as pointed out earlier - our ability to judge the minimum perfusion pressure in the individual patient which will avoid the dangers of ischaemia in every part of the diseased brain is indeed very limited today. The presence or the absence and degree of auto-regulation, vasospasm, cellular oedema, the level of anaesthesia, the choice of the anaesthetic and hypotensive drug and the technique will make the total effect on regional cerebral circulation and metabolism completely unpredictable. In many cases we witness an excellent postoperative recovery despite great difficulties during the oper-ation and anaesthesia. In other cases one despairs over a patient when an absolutely smooth and uneventful operation is followed by a more or less severe and sometimes fatal postoperative course. It is always debatable whether a certain complication was due to surgery, anaesthesia or the technique of controlled hypotension. Such dis-cussions can be instructive but are seldom conclusive.

CONCLUSIONS

It is possible that in special cases surgery is facilitated by hypotension, and that in many cases the judicious and skillful use of moderate levels of controlled hypotension will eliminate some of the risks of elective surgery. It can also be envisaged that in the near future it will be possible with the development of the monitoring de-vices mentioned above, to define in the individual patient the exact limit of pressure level below which irreversible ischaemic changes may occur. The technique of CH may then become a less controversial and more readily acceptable tool in the hands of anaesthetists.

SUMMARY

    Controlled hypotension is widely used today in neurosurgical
practice especially during the operative treatment of arterial and
arteriovenous aneurysms, where it seems to facilitate dissection and
reduce the risk of rupture and gross haemorrhage. Despite a markedly
refined technique with new drugs during recent years, controlled
hypotension still represents increased risks of cerebral ischaemia in
patients in whom loss of autoregulation, vasospasm, damage to the
blood-brain barrier and brain oedema have more or less disrupted the
normal balance between cerebral perfusion and metabolism. Before new
and more reliable monitoring devices become routinely available,
anaesthetists should therefore observe a cautious attitude to the
technique of controlled hypotension.

REFERENCES

Adams, J. H., Brierley, J. B., Conner, R. C. R., and Treip, C. S.,
        1966, The effect of systemic hypotension upon the human brain.
        Clinical and neuropathological observations in 11 cases,
        Brain, 89:235.
Astrup, J., Symon, L., Branston, N. M., and Lassen, N. A., 1977,
        Cortical evoked potentials and extracellular K^+ and H^+ at
        critical levels of brain ischemia, Stroke, 8:51.
Branston, N. M., Symon, L., Crockard, H. A., and Pasztor, E., 1974,
        Relationship between the cortical evoked potentials and local
        cortical blood flow following acute middle cerebral artery
        occlusion in the baboon, Exp.Neurol., 45:195.
Brierley, J. B., and Cooper, J. E., 1962, Cerebral complications of
        hypotensive anaesthesia in a healthy adult, J.Neurol.Neuro-
        surg.Psychiat., 25:24.
Dahlgren, B. -E., Gordon, E., and Steiner, L., 1968, Evaluation of
        controlled hypotension during surgery for intracranial arter-
        ial aneurysms, Excerpta Medica Int.Congress Series No 200,
        Proc. of the Fourth World Congress of Anaesthesiologists,
        1232.
Fein, J. M., 1975, Local cerebral oxygen extraction rates after
        middle cerebral artery occlusion, in: "Blood Flow and
        Metabolism in the Brain," M. Harper, B. Jennett, D. Miller,
        and J. Rowan, eds., Churchill-Livingstone, Edinburgh - London.
Lassen, N. A., 1980, Cerebral and spinal cord blood flow, in:
        "Anesthesia and Neurosurgery," J. E. Cottrell and H. Turndorf,
        eds., St. Louis - Toronto - London, p.1.
Lassen, N. A., and Shapiro, H. M., 1981, Anaesthesia and cerebral
        blood flow, in: "A Basis and Practice of Neuroanaesthesia,"
        E. Gordon, ed., Excerpta Medica, Amsterdam - Oxford - New
        York, p.139.
McDowall, D. G., 1981, Monitoring of electrical function as indicator
        for critical flow levels during systemic hypotension. (This
        symposium) p.

Prior, P., 1981, Critical comparison of monitoring EEG, "Cerebral
    Function" (CFM), Compressed spectral Array (CSA) and evoked
    response under conditions of reduced perfusion. (This sym-
    posium) p.
Sundt, T. M., Sharbrough, F. W., Anderson, R. E., and Michenfleder,
    J. D., 1974, Cerebral blood flow measurements and electro-
    encephalograms during carotid endarterectomy, J.Neurosurg.,
    41:310.
Symon, L., 1981, Value of cortical evoked response during neuro-
    surgical procedures. (This symposium).
Trojaborg, W., and Boysen, G., 1973, Relation between EEG, regional
    cerebral blood flow and internal carotid artery pressure
    during carotid endarterectomy, Electroenceph.Clin.Neuro-
    physiol., 34:61.

CHAIRMAN'S SUMMARY

There is a division of opinion as to whether induced hypotension
is required for neurosurgery, though the majority opinion is that
the technique is valuable. Since the main purpose of hypotension in
neurosurgery is to facilitate neurosurgical techniques, the decision
on the place of induced hypotension must be largely surgical. The
anaesthetist's role is to weigh-up, in consultation with the surgeon,
the risks compared with the benefits for any individual patient,
taking particularly into account the individual's medical history.
During the final discussion it was generally agreed that the main
hazards of induced hypotension were brain ischaemia, myocardial
ischaemia and a pre-operative history of severe hypertension. ECG
monitoring is therefore mandatory.

Once a decision has been reached that induced hypotension is
indicated for a particular operation and patient, the anaesthetist
has to consider which of the many available techniques should be
employed. In hypotension for neuroanaesthesia the two drugs most
commonly used today are sodium nitroprusside and nitroglycerine.
Both of these agents are potent cerebral vasodilators – nitroglycerine more than nitroprusside – and they therefore cause increases in intracranial blood volume and, in the closed skull, in
intracranial pressure. Nitroglycerine appears to be the less potent
agent of the two and some participants had experience of patients who
were almost totally resistant to its action. Dr. Gordon's point
about obtaining the full degree of hypotension from the beginning
with nitroglycerine and avoiding a two-stage technique of hypotension
is very relevant to this. Nitroprusside, of course, leads to cyanide
release and the recommended safe upper limit of this drug has fallen
progressively over the years. It is now believed that a total dosage
of nitroprusside of less than 1 mg/kg can produce significant cyanide

219

levels in brain and cerebro-spinal fluid. This does not mean, of course, that clinical toxicity will occur at these levels and with recent techniques of nitroprusside usage the dose levels are normally well below 1 mg/kg. The use of a vasodilator such as nitroprusside or nitroglycerine raises the possibility of steal of cerebral perfusion away from partially ischaemic zones. Remembering the concepts of thresholds of ischaemia and penumbra areas of perfusion, a vascular steal might enlarge an area of brain infarction. In my view there is still a place for trimetaphan where only moderate degrees of hypotension are required. The advantages of this drug are that it does not increase intracranial pressure and it provides an easily-controllable form of hypotension without toxicity.

The anaesthetic techniques which are used during induced hypotension in neurosurgery today include inhalational volatile agents, neurolept anaesthetic techniques and i.v. hypnotic infusions. The volatile agents halothane and (especially) enflurane can provide a useful supplementation of the hypotensive effect of any of the drugs used. However, the use of halothane or enflurane as the main hypotensive agent requires, in many patients, high dosage and therefore leads to severe reductions in cardiac output. Should an aneurysm rupture in a patient with a low cardiac output due to halothane or enflurane, resuscitation could be extremely difficult. Neurolept techniques are still popular but do not help in lowering the blood pressure. Thiopentone infusions supplement induced hypotension and, in addition, reduce brain O_2 requirements and may invoke inverse steal. However, thiopentone itself leads to prolonged post-operative drowsiness and althesin may be a suitable alternative. Yet another approach is to use 1 MAC or less of halothane or enflurane throughout the operation following opening of the dura, but to give a dose of 10-20 mg/kg thiopentone cautiously immediately before aneurysm clipping, with the object of reducing cerebral metabolism at this critical stage, and some clinicians would use larger doses still.

The beta blockers are valuable as ancillary aids in induced hypotension since they reduce the required dosage of sodium nitroprusside and avoid the tachycardia associated particularly with trimetaphan. The control of heart-rate within the range 60-80 beats/min is valuable in helping to maintain myocardial perfusion during induced hypotension. Furthermore, as Dr. Fahmys's paper demonstrated, the beta blocker drugs reduce the tendency to rebound hypertension following sodium nitroprusside but it is necessary to bear in mind their relatively short duration of action and to be ready to give further incremental doses as required.

There is still dispute about the effects of hypocapnia resulting from hyperventilation on brain perfusion levels during induced hypotension. Animal work suggests that when the blood pressure is so low as to produce critical flow conditions, all responsiveness to CO_2 is lost, so that one could argue that hypocapnia would do no harm.

However, one participant recalled a patient whose blood pressure had
been reduced to 50 mmHg systolic pressure with nitroprusside and in
whom EEG slowing occurred with hyperventilation and was reversed by
normocapnic ventilation.

The fascinating new evidence about the influence of blood glucose on the degree of brain tissue acidosis and possibly on brain
ischaemic damage suggests that patients about to undergo induced
hypotension should not have elevated blood glucose levels. However,
the normal pattern of pre-operative starvation usually ensures this
in clinical practice. The beta blockers have a glucose-lowering
effect which may be of value in this respect.

Dr. Astrup's paper reminds us of the large body of evidence
which indicates that hypothermia is the most effective technique for
brain protection. However the major practical difficulties in the
use of the technique in the course of a busy neurosurgical operating
session makes it unlikely that it will be generally accepted as a
routine for this purpose. None the less, it may still have a place
in the most difficult cases but, unfortunately, it is one of those
techniques for which regular experience is necessary to ensure safe
application. The occasional use of hypothermia may carry more hazard
to the patient than the risk of cerebral ischaemia during induced
hypotension under normothermia.

The diversity of factors in any one patient make it very difficult to know whether cerebral perfusion is adequate during induced
hypotension. Amongst these factors one might mention the surgical
pathology and the possible presence of vasospasm and/or oedema, the
presence or absence of auto-regulation, the particular drug employed
for hypotension, the possibility of steal and the depth of anaesthesia. It is therefore necessary to have some monitor of the adequacy of cerebral perfusion in the individual patient. In this
respect CBF measurement has been disappointing during operation
because of the complexity of the techniques and the lack of strictly
regional information obtained. EEG monitoring is usually impractical
because the number of electrodes necessary interfere with surgical
access. Simplified forms of EEG monitoring such as the cerebral
function monitor may have a place and Dr. Prior recommended that
during neurosurgical operations a sheet of three electrodes could be
tucked under the bone edge to provide one channel of input to the
cerebral function monitor. She pointed out, however, that this would
provide information only for the area immediately around the montor-
ing electrodes. Since in all experimental studies major reductions
in electrical activity precede brain tissue ischaemic damage, relatively simple forms of monitoring such as the cerbral function monitor give valuable information. It is doubtful whether direct cortical evoked potentials provide more information and this latter
technique has the disadvantage of being intermittent, since an evoked
potential requires about 2 min for its recording. Sensory evoked

potentials as used by Professor Symon provide additional information
concerning areas of ischaemia deep to the cortex, though again,
clinical application may be difficult and the monitoring is intermittent as discussed for direct cortical evoked potentials.

Finally, there is the problem of hypertension in the postoperative period. This can be dealt with partly by beta blockade and
partly by the use of such drugs as hydralazine. There may be oc-
casions when the blood pressure actually has to be increased following aneurysm surgery, since this may improve focal neurological
signs. The dimension of time is important here; the loss of autoregulation and the susceptibility to brain oedema secondary to surgical handling will decrease with time following surgery. The loss
of auto-regulation which follows nitroprusside hypotension probably
lasts for about one hour following the end of nitroprusside infusion.
It follows, therefore, that deliberately-induced hypertension will
have less propensity to accentuate brain oedema when used several
hours after the end of the surgical procedure.

PRINCIPAL CONTRIBUTORS

Jens Astrup, Dr.
Dept of Neurosurg
Copenhagen Country Hospital at
  Hvidovre
2650 Hvidovre
Denmark

Ulrich Braun, Prof. Dr.
Dept of Anaesthesia
Robert Koch Str 40
3400 Göttingen
FRG

James E. Cottrell, Prof. Dr.
Dept of Anesthesiology
Downstate Medical Center
State University of New York
450 Clarkson Avenue
Brooklyn
New York 11203
USA

Günther Cunitz, Prof. Dr.
Dept of Anaesthesia
Knappschafts-Krankenhaus
In der Schornau 23/25
4630 Bochum-7
FRG

Nabil R. Fahmy, Prof. Dr.
Harvard Medical School
Massachusetts General Hospital
Boston, MA 02114
USA

William Fitch, Prof. Dr.
Dept of Anaesthesia
Royal Infirmary
Glasgow G4 0SF
Scotland

Emeric Gordon, Prof. Dr.
Dept of Anaesthesia
Karolinska Hospital
10401 Stockholm
Sweden

D. I. Graham, Prof. Dr.
Univ Dept of Neuropathology
Inst of Neurol Science
Southern General Hospital
Glasgow G51 4TF
Scotland

Jürgen Grote, Prof. Dr.
Dept of Physiology
Nuballee 11
5300 Bonn
FRG

Volker Hempel, Prof. Dr.
Dept of Anaesthesia
University of Tübingen
Calwer Str. 7
D-7400 Tübingen
FRG

Dieter Heuser, Prof. Dr.
Dept of Anaesthesia
Calwer Str. 7
7400 Tübingen
FRG

Siegfried Hoyer, Prof. Dr.
Inst f Pathochemie und allg
  Neurochemie
Im Neuenheimer FEld 220-221
6900 Heidelberg-1
FRG

Klaus Huse, Prof. Dr.
Dept of Anaesthesia
Moorenstr 5
400 Düsseldorf
FRG

Hannu Kalimo, Dr.
Dept of Pathology
University of Turko
SF-20520 Turko 52
Finland

D. Gordon McDowall, Prof. Dr.
Dept of Anaesthesia
University of Leeds
24 Hyde Terrace
Leeds LS2 9LN
England

Phil J. Morris, Dr.
Dept of Anaesthesia
University of Leeds
24 Hyde Terrace
Leeds LS2 9LN
England

Thomas Pasch, Prof. Dr.
Dept of Anaesthesiology
University of Erlangen - Nürnberg
Maximilianplatz 1
D-8520 Erlangen
FRG

Volker W. A. Pickerodt, Dr.
Dept of Anaesthesia
Ev. Waldkrankenhaus
1000 Berlin-Spandau
FRG

Pamela Prior, Dr.
Consultant Clinical
  Neurophysiologist
Dept of Neurol Sciences
St Bartholomew's Hospital
West Smithfield
London EC1A 7BE
England

Stig Rehncrona, Dr.
Lab of Exp Brain Research and
  Dept of Neurosurgery
University Hospital
S-22185 Lund
Sweden

Peter J. Simpson, Dr.
University Dept of Anaesthesia
Royal Infirmary
Bristol BS2 8HW
England

Lindsay Symon, Prof. Dr.
Dept of Neurological Surgery
Inst of Neurology
Queen Square
London WC1N 3BG
England

Thomas Pasch, Prof. Dr.
Dept of Anaesthesiology
University of Erlangen – Nürnberg
Maximilianplatz 1
D-8520 Erlangen
FRG

Volker W. A. Pickerodt, Dr.
Dept of Anaesthesia
Ev. Waldkrankenhaus
1000 Berlin-Spandau
FRG

Pamela Prior, Dr.
Consultant Clinical
  Neurophysiologist
Dept of Neurol Sciences
St Bartholomew's Hospital
West Smithfield
London EC1A 7BE
England

Stig Rehncrona, Dr.
Lab of Exp Brain Research and
  Dept of Neurosurgery
University Hospital
S-22185 Lund
Sweden

Peter J. Simpson, Dr.
University Dept of Anaesthesia
Royal Infirmary
Bristol BS2 8HW
England

Lindsay Symon, Prof. Dr.
Dept of Neurological Surgery
Inst of Neurology
Queen Square
London WC1N 3BG
England

Acetylcholine, 95
  synthesis, 95, 101
Acidosis, 71
  extracellular, 72
ADH, 26
ADP, 185
Afterload, 21
Alpha receptors, 13
Althesin, 193, 194, 195
AMP, 185
Amplitude measure (EEG), 124
Aneurysms, cerebral arterial, 79
Aneurysm surgery, 31, 125, 133,
     212
Angiotensin
  I, 14, 26
  II, 12, 14, 26
  III, 26
  antagonism, 14
Angiotensinogen, 26
Apoplectic patients, 71
Arterio-venous malformations, 212
ATP, 63, 85
  generation, 72, 76
Autoregulation, 59, 61, 120, 121,
     129, 204, 205

Barbiturate, 87, 89
Berg Fourier analyzer, 123
Blockade
  alpha-, 4, 5, 12
  beta-, 4, 5
Blood flow, regional, 181
Boundary zones, brain damage in,
     120, 121, 164, 165
Bradykinin, 28

Brain
  perfusion pressure, 160, 164
  protection, 63, 89
Brainstem herniation, 152
Burst suppression, 118

Calcium channel blockers, 52
Cardiac
  arrest, 158, 165
  output 4, 5, 22, 23, 52
Cardiopulmonary bypass, 86
Carotid artery occlusion, 98,
     119, 121
Carotid artery occlusion,
     unilateral, 65
Catecholamines, 12, 23
Cerebral
  blood flow, 32, 53, 59, 60, 61,
     86, 100, 117
  electric activity, 119
  function analyzer monitor
     (CFAM), 126
  function monitor (CFM), 114,
     124, 126, 214
  glucose uptake (CMRgluc), 86,
     99, 100
  ischemia, 114
  oxygen uptake (CMRO$_2$), 53, 86,
     99, 100
  perfusion pressure (CPP), 32,
     52, 93, 97, 145, 149
Cholinesterases, 42
Clipping of artery, 73
Collateral blood supply, 162
Compressed spectral array (CSA),
     114, 117, 123

Conduction time, central somato-
        sensory (CTT), 114, 122
Controlled hypotension (CH):
        indication, 212
Coronary artery disease, 206
Curare, 4, 5
Cyanide, 7, 50

Density modulated spectral array
        (DSA), 123
Diazoxide, 35
Dilators, arteral and venous, 49
Doppler, 121

ECG, 195
EEG, 113, 117, 121, 123, 124, 214
Electron microscopy, 172-177
Enflurane, 32, 33, 34, 145
Epidural or spinal anesthesia, 4
Etomidate, 74
Evoked response, evoked
        potentions, 114, 117,
        118, 119, 121, 122, 126,
        214
    (see also Somatosensory evoked
        potentials (SEP))
Extracellular fluid, 80, 82

Fentanyl, 43, 194, 196
Fick's principle, 204
Fourier transformation, 123
Focal hypoxic brain damage, 158

Ganglion blockage, 4, 5, 12
Ganglionic blocking drugs, 49
Glucose, 71
    metabolism, 94
Glycolytic blockers, 64

H^+-activity, 72
Halothane, 4, 12, 32, 33, 60, 165
Heart rate, 193
Hexamethonium, 4
Hydralyzin, 35
Hydrogen clearance, 83
Hyperglycemia, 71, 74
Hypertension, 119, 165
    rebound arterial, 21, 27, 28,
        50
Hyperventilation, 204
    (see also Hypocapnia)

Hypocapnia, arterial, 185
Hypoglycemia, 71
Hypothermia, 85, 90
Hypoxemia, 94
Hypoxia
    normocapnic, 182
    several types combined, 166
Hypoxic vascular response,
        pulmonary, 44

Interactions, drug, 41
Intermittent positive pressure
        ventilation, 4
Intracranial pressure, 6, 51,
        145-152
Ion leak fluxes, 85
Ischemia
    cerebral, 71
    complete, 171
    incomplete, 64, 171, 172
    incomplete regional, 72
Ischemic
    brain damage, 118-120, 158, 171
    nerve cell change, 158,
        172
    threshold time, 164

Juxtaglomerular apparatus, cells,
        26

K^+-electrode, 72, 80
Krypton 85, 80, 83

Labeltalol, 4
Lactacidosis, 65, 71, 72, 76, 98,
        172-176
Lactate, 64, 65, 66, 94
    /pyruvate-ratio, 187
Lidocaine, 85, 86, 90
Light microscopy, 172

MAC, 33
Mean arterial blood pressure, 164
Membrane
    failure, 63
    stabilization, 76, 85, 88
Methaemoglobin, 7
Methoxyflurane, 32
Microelectrodes, ion-selective,
        72

Middle cerebral artery, 72, 73
Monitoring, routine, 52
Muscle relaxants, 41, 43, 44

Neostigmine, 45
Nitroglycerine
  tri-nitroglycerine (TNG), 4-17,
    41, 51, 61
  glyceryl trinitrate (GTN), 145,
    146
Nitroprusside, 4-17, 21-28, 61,
    114
  (*see also* Sodium-nitroprusside)
Normoglycemia, 71

Ohm's law, 203
Oxidative brain metabolism, 93
Oxygen
  consumption, cerebral, 95
  (*see also* Cerebral Oxygen
    uptake)
  tension, 181, 184, 185
  uptake ($\dot{V}O_2$), 204

pCO_2, 4, 93, 94, 98
Pentobarbital, 87
Pentolinium, 4, 5, 12
Penumbra flow concept, 114
Penumbral zone, 214
Period-amplitude display, 126
Pharmacokinetics, 42
Phenoxybenzamine, 4, 5
Phentolamine, 4, 5, 13
Phosphocreatinine, 181, 185
Phosphofructokinase, 185
Plasma protein binding, 42
Potassium
  extracellular, 86
  release, 71, 73, 76
Practolol, 4, 81
Preload, 21
Pressure
  /flow relationship, 60, 61
  right atrial, 22
Propanidid, 42
Propranolol, 4, 21, 23, 34
Prostaglandins, 28
Pyruvate, 94

Recovery, postischemic, 65. 67
Regional blood flow, 213
  (*see also* Cerebral regional
    blood flow CBFr)
Regional cerebral blood flow
  (rCBF), 54
Renal perfusion, 42
Renin, 21-28, 51
Renin-angiotensin-system, 21, 26,
    34
Rhodanese, 7

Saralasin, 28
Sensory evoked potentials (SEP),
    114
  (*see also* Evoked potentials)
Sodium nitroprusside (SNP), 4-17,
    21, 41, 50, 79, 80, 81,
    82, 84, 145
  (*see also* Nitroprusside)
Space-occupying lesion (SOL),
    145, 146
Stagnant hypoxia, 157, 158, 161
  (*see also* Ischemia)
Subarachnoid hemorrhage, 6
Succinylcholine, 42
Swan-Ganz-catheter, 209

Thiocyanate, 7, 43, 50
Thiopental, 86
Thiosulfate, 44
Threshold of ischemia, 165
Trimethaphan (TMP), 4, 12, 34,
    41, 42, 51, 79, 80

Urapidil, 13, 35

Vascular smooth muscle cells, 11
Vasodilators, direct acting, 6,
    14
Vitamin B_{12}, 7, 43, 44
Volatile anesthetics, 31

133-Xenon, 60